Studying Nursing Using Problem-Based and Enquiry-Based Learning

Studying Nursing Using Problem-Based and Enquiry-Based Learning

Bob Price

palgrave
macmillan

First published 2003 by
PALGRAVE MACMILLAN
Houndmills, Basingstoke, Hampshire RG21 6XS and
175 Fifth Avenue, New York, N.Y. 10010
Companies and representatives throughout the world

PALGRAVE MACMILLAN is the global academic imprint of the Palgrave Macmillan division of St. Martin's Press, LLC and of Palgrave Macmillan Ltd. Macmillan® is a registered trademark in the United States, United Kingdom and other countries. Palgrave is a registered trademark in the European Union and other countries.

ISBN-13: 978-0-333-98414-7
ISBN-10: 0-333-98414-5

Logging, pulping and manufacturing processes are expected to conform to the environmental regulations of the country of origin.
This book is printed on paper suitable for recycling and made from fully managed and sustained forest sources.

A catalogue record for this book is available from the British Library.

Printed and bound by CPI Antony Rowe, Eastbourne

This textbook is dedicated to students of nursing and those who help them learn how to think and think how to change. It is also dedicated to Adrienne and to James, my own family teachers.

CONTENTS

LIST OF TABLES

List of Boxes

LIST OF FIGURES

INTRODUCTION

Pause for a moment to consider what much of nursing practice consists of and you might reasonably conclude that it is enquiry and problem-solving. We solve problems with, and sometimes for, patients. When we are not directly engaged in problem-solving, we are often involved in making inquiries so those problems can be solved. Much of the work that nurses do in public health, health promotion or primary care is associated with helping others either to avoid or minimize problems as part of lifestyle maintenance. It is perhaps not surprising, then, that during the past five years there has been a growth in problem-based and enquiry-based learning approaches (PBL/EBL) within nurse education. If nurses are first and foremost 'knowledge workers', using their knowledge to help others and assisting patients to acquire and use knowledge for themselves, it is important that they are educated as critical thinkers, able to manage information effectively. The collection, analysis and application of knowledge are at the centre of problem-solving. Problem-solving is a complex skill involving assessment of the situation, recognition of what is known or of that, which is not yet understood, and inquiry designed to gather relevant information. Problem-solving usually involves working closely with others precisely because one professional working alone does not easily solve problems. Nurse teachers have been quick to realize the merits of teaching nurses problem-solving skills within the nursing curriculum. In some instances, problem- or enquiry-based learning is the preferred learning approach for a whole syllabus. In other cases, problem-based learning is employed within particular modules of study.

This textbook is for nurses who are interested in learning about solving problems or understanding practice using modern means of education. It is written from the student perspective, assisting you with the process of learning through problem- or enquiry-based approaches. It is of particular relevance to students enrolled upon nurse education programmes where PBL or EBL provides the curriculum framework, but is also relevant for nurses who decide to use these approaches for their own professional update. Because problem-solving practice is a co-operative and inquisitive form of learning and practice adjustment, it is well suited to groups of nurses who wish to work together to improve practice within their own area. The chapters are written with both learner audiences in mind – those completing a nurse education programme, and those setting out in a collegiate group to improve nursing practice beyond that.

This textbook is not primarily intended for education programme designers. These colleagues already have a number of resources open to them. Nevertheless, this text does provide a range of material, associated with working in groups, liaising with a facilitator and preparing for project closure and/or assessment that will make this a useful reference for tutors and those clinical experts who might mentor nurses making PBL or EBL inquiries.

THE LAYOUT OF THIS BOOK

The text is arranged in three Parts. It has been designed so as to represent an informative resource when read completely and thereafter as an important reference that might be dipped into on an individual chapter basis. Parts II and III in particular provide useful information on specific aspects of learning using problem- and enquiry-based approaches, and illustrate the form such inquiries might take. If you are unfamiliar with problem- or enquiry-based learning I recommend that you read the book through first and then return to the relevant chapters during the course of your studies. If you are already a confident learner, using problem-solving practice methods, then you may care to start with Part III first and compare the inquiries there with your own experience. Looking back through Part II will help you understand how those projects were conducted, and why they arrived at the solutions that they did!

Practice and learning

Part I of the textbook is entitled 'Practice and Learning'. It sets out the premises that underpin this textbook and much of the problem-based learning teaching that I have employed to date. Briefly put, these are that nursing practice is usually challenging and requires the thoughtful application of knowledge in order to arrive at actions that seem relevant and helpful. Nursing theory and health care research, on their own, do not transform practice for the better. Instead, nurses need to learn to combine different elements, fitting them to problems and challenges, so that solutions might be found. The synthesis of different forms of information, from different sources, within the context of a particular need is greatly enhanced when you employ a problem-solving framework or approach. The purpose of learning is not only utilitarian (assisting the client), it is developmental. If you learn to analyse and then solve problems, to make further inquiries as part of a group, you will be better equipped to become a lifelong learner and to improve your own practice.

To this end, Chapter 1 explains just why practice is often complex or problematical and why, even after a course of studies, you will need to remain an inquisitive practitioner. It is important to understand what we mean by problem-based learning (Chapter 2) and enquiry-based learning (Chapter 3). While PBL and EBL approaches share some common assumptions (for instance, they both emphasize learning conducted with others), they also involve subtle differences. A case is made in Part I for distinguishing between the two, because if you embark upon a particular form of study you need to understand the approach you are using. The more you understand the principles of what you are doing, the less likely you are to lose your way within projects.

Chapter 4 offers information on a scaffold with which to understand the different fields of inquiry that might be explored as part of PBL or EBL. If you are reading this textbook in association with a PBL/EBL programme of studies, then it is likely that you will already have been provided with a basic introduction to the approach. In most instances this has been drawn either from the experience of colleagues using PBL curricula in North America, or through that of colleagues educating others within Europe (especially The Netherlands). For those readers who are using this textbook for professional update, however, it is useful to provide a scaffold with which to plan your inquiries. This does not replace the principles of problem- or enquiry-based learning, but it does cover some of the most common dimensions of problems that you are likely to encounter. For example, problems might arise concerning knowledge (gaps in knowledge – lack of relevance or inappropriate foci), decision-making, evidence for practice or philosophy (how professionals approach practice situations and understand their role and goals). You should find these problem dimensions useful, irrespective of your study context.

Making inquiries

Part II forms by far the largest portion of this textbook and represents a journey through the process of conducting your own inquiries. Successful problem- or enquiry-based learning is founded upon assessing the nature of the practice situation and then accessing appropriate information from a variety of sources. We need to understand what is problematic about a situation, why it seems problematic, in order to generate 'learning issues'. Once these have been identified, this suggests the need for additional information and/or guidance. Chapters 5 and 6 of this book explain the process of acquiring new information from different sources. Chapter 5 attends to gathering information from clinical, library, and human expert sources. Chapter 6 focuses specifically upon the World Wide Web. The Internet provides a massive fund of potential new knowledge but it does require practice to access it and also wisdom to use it. Not everything you discover on the web is either authoritative or impartial!

Once you have discovered new information, it has to be evaluated and incorporated within your analysis. It is important at this stage to work effectively with group members and to make the very best use of your group facilitator. Chapter 7 discusses this process, highlighting some of the challenges and the ways forward for conducting a useful analysis of the problem. You are then in a position to plan a new round of action, perhaps new lines of inquiry, or the preparation of a solution to the problem identified.

In any PBL/EBL project there eventually comes the moment when the project must reach closure (Chapter 8). If the project has been completed as part of a programme of studies, then there is often an assessment to be prepared for. Chapter 9 discusses these matters, and shows not only ways to represent what you have learned, but the means by which to evaluate how the inquiry was undertaken. Real-life problems, within the clinical field, often cannot be resolved in the short term. We learn to make incremental progress, and to examine whether our goals were ambitious or clear.

Two case studies

The final two chapters within this book are presented in Part III. Chapter 10 offers an illustration of a problem-based learning inquiry, while Chapter 11 provides an example from enquiry-based learning. The aim of these chapters is not to present an ideal, but to demonstrate the course of inquiry that led to a particular outcome. The case studies are not exemplary, or unproblematic. They represent much that is good and some that did not go according to plan. Students often report that it is difficult to understand the direction that an inquiry is taking, or to manage the anxieties associated with inquiries when they are in the midst of these. There can be no simple template for projects, but these illustrations do provide an overview of the decisions, directions and refinement of thinking that are a mark of problem- and enquiry-based learning in progress.

Finally, at the back of this book you will find a glossary of key terms. Like any other educational approach, problem- and enquiry-based learning approaches have developed a terminology of their own. To assist you with this I set out the most important terms as they are used within this textbook and with reference to how they have sometimes been employed elsewhere.

Part I

PRACTICE AND LEARNING

1 THE NATURE OF HEALTH CARE PROBLEMS AND PRACTICE

We live in a world where there are many alternative accounts of what represents 'best practice'. We deliver nursing care at a time when the consumer may be tempted to take legal proceedings because health care has not been as they imagined it *should* be. Nursing today is a public performance profession. You almost certainly deliver care within the public eye. It is important to make the best decisions and to work sensitively with the patient and lay carers. The successful nurse is the sensitive nurse. He or she understands not only the theory behind different techniques, but also when it is wise to employ such techniques (Penny and Warelow, 1999). Nurses today not only need to be knowledgeable and skilful, they need to be wise (Bradshaw, 2001).

Twenty or so years ago the nature of nursing was rather more straightforward (Kershaw, 1998). If you went into the nursing care library and took out a book, it was likely to be arranged under medical headings. There would be sections on medical and surgical nursing. Significantly, nursing action would be described in terms of a response to a disease or treatment. There was a formula for asthma care, for post-operative nursing and for managing the care of a head-injured patient. Look back through textbooks of the time and it is easy to become nostalgic. Nursing was less complicated. Nurses followed the directions of medical colleagues and it was possible to list what you did in any given situation. Those who marked assignment questions then knew full well that they could rely upon a limited list of 'things to be demonstrated' before the answer was judged passworthy.

Practice is not like that today though. If you have just begun studying nursing, or are perhaps completing a post-registration course, it is quickly apparent that finding the right answers,

9

saying the right thing, offering the right care are no longer quite
so easy (Price, 1998a). Going on a clinical placement can prove
daunting precisely because whatever you have read does not
quite seem to fit with the reality of care-giving. When you walk
onto a ward it's not simply that you must learn a wealth of
information, it is that you must understand how others, the
patients and your colleagues think (Morales-Mann and Kaitell,
2001). Practice involves understanding people, as well as processes and procedures (Wheeler, 2001; Wong *et al.*, 2001). We
have to learn how to 'read' situations and even how to decide
whether what we have seen or heard is significant (Price, B.,
2001a; Rundio, 2001). When you come to think about it, one of
the greatest skills you will learn as a nurse is how to decide
whether something is problematic in the first place! This is no
idle muse. Health care resources are limited so we must prioritize
care and tackle what are sometimes called the priority problems.
Identifying what needs our further attention is therefore key to
strategic practice.

Within problem- and enquiry-based learning, the nature of
the situation, that which might be problematic, is assumed to be
unclear. Problems are not always apparent or readily labelled. It
is unrealistic therefore to start this book with an instant explanation of every problem that might occur in practice. What is
important, however, is to begin with a discussion of what might
represent some of the characteristics of problems. This not only
informs how or why nurses and others have to investigate practice,
but it also explains why nurses need to be consummate inquirers
and problem-solvers. It is this which has changed so fundamentally within nursing. Today we need to interpret practice for
ourselves. The instant formulas or theories have gone and many
in any case were poor guides to practice. It is apparent that the
traditional way of learning (hear a theory – apply a theory – check
whether it worked) is no longer enough. At best, practitioners
are left wondering why theory did not seem to fit practice. At
worst, they try to make practice fit the theory.

WHAT IS A PROBLEM?

Nurses often describe themselves as helpers and problem-solvers
(Erdmann, 1998). This begs the fundamental question, just what

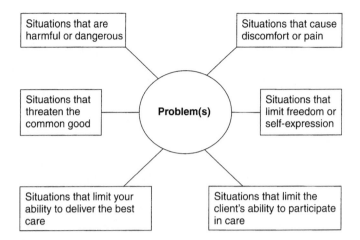

Figure 1.1   The nature of problems

is a problem? In Figure 1.1 I itemize some of the reasons why something (perhaps a health care situation or a future course of action) might be construed as a problem. When you look at this diagram it is worth asking yourself an additional question. Who defines the problem?

There are many situations where the nurse identifies behaviour or environmental factors that represent a threat to the health or well-being of clients. Penicillin-resistant strains of bacteria, asbestos fibres within a working environment or smoking cigarettes are but a few examples. In these circumstances it is often quite difficult to agree who defines the problem, naming the situation or threat as 'problematic'. For example, even today some employers refuse to acknowledge legal liability for asbestosis, mesothelioma and other illnesses associated with the exposure of workers to asbestos dust. In these contexts there may be relatively few debates about the causation of illness or damage, but there may arise complex arguments about who was responsible for the threat, and at what level something (asbestos dust, cigarettes) become harmful.

Most people would consider something that caused discomfort or pain to be problematic. Surgery, chemotherapy treatment for cancer or group therapy used to tackle unsociable behaviour are all potentially problematic for the patient. They may, however, also be therapeutic. That is, they may offer benefits to the patient. Nurses often recommend the worth of dealing with short-term treatment discomfort to achieve longer-term ends. The nurse provides anti-emetics to help the patient cope with nausea after administration of cytotoxic drugs. She helps to counter the problem that she has herself contributed to. In such situations nurses and patients try to redefine the threat as acceptable, tolerable or worthwhile. It may, for example, be worth putting up with some hair loss to protect health in the longer term.

Many ethical problems associated with practice concern the rights of individuals and the rights of groups (Inglis, 2000; Burckhardt, 2002). Consider the situation of a nurse who is HIV positive (Human Immunodeficiency Virus) and who understandably wishes to lead a lifestyle that he considers valuable and professional. Against this, however, there are others within the local community who have misgivings about being treated by such a practitioner and moreover who suggest that 'HIV Positive people' should have their names recorded upon a register and then have their professional freedom restricted in some way. Problems are not always open to simple definition. One person's normality is another person's problem. Within health care you will meet situations where people cannot agree whether something is problematic. In practice, some problems are personally defined in terms of values, attitudes and experiences. It can be very difficult for us to understand the problems of others, or perhaps to empathize with their position.

The organization of health care itself can be problematic where it limits the ability of the patient to make decisions about and participate in his or her own care. Historically health care professions have defined their contribution on the basis of expertize and the holding of a unique body of knowledge. Sometimes this knowledge is complex. Sometimes it is portrayed as complex because the health care professional wishes to retain control over decision-making. Tilley and colleagues, however, emphasize that nurses should help empower patients (Tilley et al., 1999). However, tensions can and do arise in chronic illnesses where patients research their own conditions and then challenge health care professionals on the best way forward. It can be challenging to help patients and lay carers feel part of a rehabilitation or care plan (Yates, 1997). Problems therefore are frequently associated with power. That includes the power to define what is problematic in the first place and, thereafter, the power to define what should be done about it.

Problems exist for nurses as much as they do for patients. Consider the scenario where you have completed a literature review on wound care and where you have amassed a substantial body of research evidence that suggests a particular wound care technique delays rather than hastens healing. When you deliver your findings to medical and senior nurse colleagues, they acknowledge that the results are intriguing, but elect to continue with their chosen practice because they feel that further evidence is required before a new protocol can be established. Problems exist therefore where there are differences of vision or goal and where there may also be disagreement regarding the best means to achieve a goal. Health care often involves debates about what *should* be done, or supported. This is not necessarily a scientific debate. Health care professionals have their own and collective ideologies (Traynor, 1999; Browne, 2001). That is, they try to define what is normal, preferable, appropriate, expert or aesthetic (Woodall, 2000). Where individuals challenge such ideologies, a problem may arise for all parties concerned – the change agent and those supporting the status quo. In these situations the nurse's challenge itself becomes defined as problematic, because it questions what is understood to be the common good of the team.

So what can we now say about the nature of health care problems? Box 1.1 sums up what may be the characteristics of a problem.

Box 1.1   The characteristics of problems

- The origin, parameters or components of the problem may be hotly contested (what caused what?, why did this happen?, what do we need to consider here?).
- Problems may be contextual. What is problematic in one environment may not be so in another.
- Problems have a scale (this may refer to the level of risk, the volume of work or skill needed to rectify the problem).
- Problems may sometimes be necessary. It may, relatively speaking, be necessary to create one problem in order to solve a larger one.

Box 1.1   (continued)

- Problems are often personally defined and may be ideological or attitude and value-related.
- Others' problems are sometimes difficult to discern or to empathize with.
- The problem may be as much about agreeing ways to respond to a situation as they are about the situation itself. Problems are therefore open to escalation when an opening problem (definition agreed) is tackled in ways that are not universally supported.
- Problems may sometimes be unresolvable. That is, interested parties may not be able to agree the best solution or the preferred solution may be unattainable. In some situations patients and nurses have to 'live with the problem', accepting a new state of affairs. In such circumstances the situation may be redefined as unproblematic in order to deal with the tensions posed by having failed to change the situation.

IS HEALTH CARE MORE PROBLEMATIC TODAY?

You may agree with many other nurses that nursing practice is more stressful today and that this is associated with the volume and complexity of problems that you tackle at work. While it would be difficult to quantify the volume of problems faced by nurses at different times, anecdotally it does seem likely that practice is experienced as more problematic today. A wide variety of situations and expectations can be conceived as problematic and prompt you to try and change matters (see Figure 1.2). The more the public and health care professionals consider health or illness in problem terms (as something worthy of investigation and resolution) the more important problem solving skills become.

While problems can simply occur (for instance, associated with physical deterioration in old age), they can also be made. Look at the following short studies, which demonstrate this point:

> Mrs Joyce is admitted to hospital for hip replacement surgery. She is 78 years old and obese. Surgical techniques, improvements in

anaesthetics and nursing support measures such as the use of anti-embolism stockings mean that treatment is likely to be effective. Having read about the risks of hospital-acquired infections, however, her daughter is eager that Mrs Joyce is discharged as quickly as possible. This will require careful liaison and regular visits by community staff to ensure that her progress remains satisfactory.

Louise is a recently qualified midwife who is committed to the philosophy of woman-centred care and the promotion of natural childbirth as far as this is professionally possible. She suffers a number of uncomfortable encounters with other midwives and obstetricians whom she sees as 'interventionist'. These colleagues assess the risk to the woman and the importance of her birth aspirations differently. They recommend intervening sooner and often more radically. As a result, there are sometimes arguments in the labour suite.

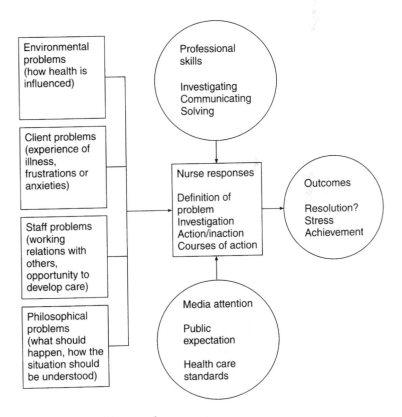

Figure 1.2 Problems and responses

In the first of these examples part of the problem relates to public expectations. Patients expect more services than in the past and that these are conducted to the highest standards. In previous decades, Mrs Joyce may have been excluded from surgery simply because we could not contain the risks effectively. As health care has improved, so more elderly patients are undergoing bigger operations and achieving greater levels of mobility and comfort. Surgery solves a problem (hip pain and immobility) but expectations associated with it cause other problems. How will Mrs Joyce be supported within the community? How in the interim will we minimize the risk that this vulnerable patient does not contract a hospital-based infection? As Mrs Joyce and other patients live longer, thanks in part to health care treatment, how can we ensure that they receive adequate care in their homes where they would prefer to remain?

The second problem is also manufactured. In this instance, competing ideologies of midwifery care clash in the context of the delivery suite. There are debates about cases that were 'problematic'. Did these illustrate Louise's reluctance to read the warning signs and to agree timely intervention? Alternatively, was Louise's stance correct, holding out and working with the mother to achieve a natural birth, until such time that it became clear that a Caesarean section was unavoidable? If professional colleagues cannot agree a protocol for practice, can they agree means of mutually assessing risk to a client? Is it possible to negotiate parameters beyond which everyone agrees that additional intervention is necessary?

What appears to make health care practice seem more problematic therefore is not only the volume and range of needs and expectations presented by the public, but that the solutions to these problems must be robust. Women having babies desire a natural childbirth but also a process that is ideally also fail-safe. It is then difficult to achieve a balance between these two expectations when there are different recommendations regarding what represents good practice. Nurses and midwives have to make the best possible decisions under time constraints and with finite amounts of knowledge. Standards of practice are widely publicized and equally the scare stories are highlighted within the media. There is greater accountability for practice at a time when, increasingly, society as well as the professions debate what equals best practice.

Not only is health care practice more problematic, but it is also more problem-orientated. We are much more likely to define situations as problematic. This is partly because we are cautious about how others, especially consumers, will interpret practice, but also because there is a wider diversity of opinion on how to proceed. Science has made us more aware of what could happen and society has reminded us of the penalties that health care organizations might now have to pay if the best decisions were not made.

THE NEED FOR THE INQUISITIVE PRACTITIONER

Circumstances such as those described above make it clear that the practitioner has to be inquisitive and clearly aware of what is to be achieved. That is, we need to be reflexive practitioners (White, 1999). We cannot assume the definition of what is happening nor that other interested parties will see health care as we do. Theorists explain that this is because we live within what has been described as a postmodernist society (Theodore, 1998). We are part of a society where there are many norms for behaviour, many different ideas about what would seem best to do and at a time when people are increasingly encouraged to challenge the view of experts in whatever field they operate. Everyone has an opinion, so it becomes important to understand the different viewpoints when dealing with something as important and intimate as health care.

Studying nursing at university you are very likely to be taught skills of reflection, critical thinking and problem analysis for precisely these reasons (Brookfield, 1987; Milligan, 1999). These are transferable skills that not only help you to address practice needs now, but to go on doing so in the years after you have left the lecture theatre (Gopee, 2000). Arguably, nurses need transferable skills, those associated with inquiry and communication now more than ever before (Bjornsdottir, 2000). The ability to find out and to contribute to accounts of problems and their possible resolution is key to helping you manage the stress of professional life (Dobson *et al.*, 2000). A successful problem investigator is likely to be a practitioner who also gains satisfaction from practice and who feels that he or she is making a worthwhile contribution.

Imagine for a moment what this means in practice. Let's assume that you are interviewing a elderly man who is being admitted to hospital with chest problems. It is clear that his breathing is laboured and that he finds it difficult to give a health history. He looks exhausted and you notice a bluish tinge to his face, which suggests that he is cyanosed, struggling to get oxygen around his body. This patient is accompanied by his wife who is clearly anxious about the situation and who does her best to answer most of your questions on behalf of her husband. As she intervenes with answers you realize that she is partially deaf. She has misunderstood what you were asking. Flicking through the case notes that have arrived with the patient you see that a provisional medical diagnosis of emphysema related to smoking has been made. You look up and smile at the couple resting before you. The problem before you is not simply the medical diagnosis of emphysema. It is how to assist this couple most sensitively and effectively. What will you do first? How will you make the patient comfortable? When is it better to reserve history taking until later? Has the gentlemen's wife really got a hearing problem or might you have posed your questions in too complex a way?

This scenario is relatively common. It is not an emergency nor is it exceptional. When you cast your mind back to the textbooks and lectures you recall that there was information on chest illnesses, on health assessment, on communication skills and upon anxiety and its impact upon health and comprehension of situations. Your greatest wish might be to have a definitive answer to this conundrum – what shall I do first and why? In practice, however, what makes this situation quite unlike the textbooks is that you must decide how to mix the different information you have. How do you combine the knowledge available so that it serves this patient and his wife best?

It can be extremely tempting to resolve the situation by prematurely defining it in one or more ways. It is certainly more comfortable to think of the patient as emphysemic and his wife as simply anxious. But these are labels that might not tell the whole story when we pause to consider what represents good nursing care. They may be sufficient to tackle some of the greatest threats (for instance, associated with oxygen depletion), but they hardly address the patient's experience of illness. We need to place this episode within the context of the patient's world. What does dyspnoea represent to him? Yes, it is frightening, but does it also become associated with guilt? Perhaps later the patient confides that he feels foolish having smoked cigarettes all his life. He feels a burden on his wife and now on the hard-pressed health care services.

To deliver sensitive care it will be necessary to inquire further into the experience of illness and hospital admission. It may be necessary to investigate the care implications when it is discovered that the patient suffers not only from emphysema but also diabetes mellitus. That may mean that you need to reread textbooks, to look at recent research papers, to discuss the health care assessment with the consultant and to debate with the dietician and physiotherapist what represents the best package of rehabilitation in the next weeks. It will be important to know how to find out information and to use this in a particular context. At first, it will be necessary to know where to look for information and what questions should be asked. All of this stems from the nature of the problem that has emerged.

When we pause to consider what is different within this practice it is that we must learn to work in two ways (see Figure 1.3). We need to become expert gatherers of information from the situation before us. We need to make what Eraut (1990) has called 'tacit knowledge' apparent to all of our colleagues by talking about what we see or hear. This helps us shape the questions that we ask and the sort of additional information or guidance that might help us respond most effectively. Equally, we need to become good at analysing accounts of problems, the explanations that others offer regarding what is happening or why it is happening. We need therefore to unpick what the explanations mean. What does it mean, for instance, to be cyanosed? What does it mean to be anxious? When we combine work with information from both sources, the situation and the theories or accounts, we are likely to produce better answers.

Problem- and enquiry-based learning approaches are techniques designed to help you develop the sort of inquisitive skills that work well in situations such as those described above. They not only help you to manage a patient's admission to hospital in a sensitive way, but also help you to understand why other practitioners hold strong views upon health care issues such as childbirth. They help to explain why working in health care can seem stressful and can prompt new ways to feel professional in the face of considerable demands and pressures.

Learning how to make inquiries or to solve problems involves learning how to think and work inductively and deductively.

Reading the situation, using our eyes and ears, the questions and tests that we run.	→	Deciding what this means. What do we need to do? What else do we need to learn?	→	Forming a working theory or account of what is going on (tentative at first).

Inductive work

The nurse 'reads' the patient's face and concludes that the blue appearance means that he is cyanosed. Poor supply of oxygen makes mobility difficulty and may impair thinking. This patient may not be well placed to give a health history right now.

Anxiety interferes with our ability to interpret situations – we may react abruptly or defensively.	→	The hospital is a stressful place. It is a new environment.	→	I need to proceed sympathetically and to expect that he or she might 'snap'.

Deductive work

The nurse has a theory which, whilst not necessarily a perfect fit for the situation, could illuminate why the patient's wife behaves as she does. It is used to understand why she is tense and asks questions so sharply. As a result, the nurse reacts thoughtfully, helping the wife to cope with her sudden feelings.

Figure 1.3   Ways of working with information

It teaches you how to combine the two processes. Reflection is not always enough (Taylor, 2001). Simply applying theory from a textbook rarely works. It is the combination of theory and reflection, within the context of a group effort, that makes the fundamental difference to how you operate. I hope that this chapter has set the scene for such learning and convinced you that there is personal benefit in learning using PBL and EBL techniques. They are not simply an educational quirk or a new way of teaching. At their very best they can help transform the way in which you think and work at the bedside! Completed successfully with the help of a facilitator, they can represent the very best means of becoming a confident and then later an expert practitioner of nursing.

2 PROBLEM-BASED LEARNING

Wilkie (2000, p. 11) describes problem-based learning as an 'instructional method in which students work in small groups to gain knowledge and acquire problem-solving skills. A major characteristic of PBL is that the problem is presented to the student *before* the material has been learned rather than after.' This could seem rather a daunting prospect, but it does have the merit that it mimics the reality of clinical practice. A 'dollop of explanatory theory' does not helpfully precede patients who walk through the door of your surgery, or come attached to problems that arise within practice contexts. As practitioners we have to make sense of the situation as it develops, to learn to read what is happening and what therefore might be needed in the future. In these regards, nursing work, like police work, is investigative in nature.

HISTORICAL ROOTS

It is useful to understand the origins of problem-based learning because you can then compare the situation that prompted their development then with that relating to nursing today. Problem-based learning emerged as an approach because there was considered to be a significant gap between what was taught in the classroom and what was required in the practice setting. Problem-based learning has its historical origins within medical education in North America and subsequently Western Europe (Schmidt, 1983; Neufeld *et al.*, 1989; Price, 1998a). Educators identified a fundamental problem in the training of doctors. Medical students were taught significant volumes of theory, before they ventured into clinical areas, where they were required to translate abstract concepts into practice and to apply the reasoning that had been illustrated within the classroom. Not only did this involve students in trying to identify what among their learning was most significant, but to match relevant teaching to the vague and complicated problems or histories that the patients presented with. There was no guarantee that what students had been taught within the classroom would become quickly relevant with the first medical 'cases' that they encountered. Moreover, the students quickly observed that the theoretical skills they learned on university campus did not match those that more experienced doctors used in practice. To draw a simple analogy – medical practitioners built jigsaws without the aid of a picture on the box, while the medical students had been provided with a variety of jigsaw pictures that might not be relevant to the puzzles they were meant to solve.

Barrows and others (Barrows and Tamblyn, 1980) proposed that, instead of assisting doctors with their clinical skills, large volumes of pre-clinical teaching inhibited their ability to think in ways that were clinically important. The theories explained in college constrained the students' understanding of health and illness, and therefore there was merit in reversing the process. Instead of presenting students first with theories to be tested out subsequently in practice, they should be presented with problems that encouraged them to theorize about what was happening for themselves. This, in practice, was what practitioners had to do, drawing selectively upon some existing knowledge, and adding to that with new knowledge (e.g. medical investigations) in order to make a diagnosis and prepare a plan of treatment.

Medical ethics prevented educators from exposing live patients to the students' untutored problem-solving investigations. Medical education, like nurse education, had to ensure that learning was not achieved at the expense of patient safety. For this reason, Barrows proposed that the medical curriculum should be devised around a series of patient situations that were drawn from real clinical situations, but which were presented to the students as cases away from the ward. Case notes came with challenges attached (Barrows, 1986). Different patient problems would be presented so as to acknowledge students' learning to date, to fit with subjects within the curriculum and to encourage the development of particular clinical skills (e.g. history taking). Some information would be presented with the scenario, but other information would be missing. Students were then challenged to assess what the problem consisted of, what they already knew and might be counted as fact, what they did not yet understand or know, or therefore would need to be found out from a variety of sources (Price, B., 2000a).

Problem-based learning was therefore conceived as inquisitive, and requiring students to gather, sift and analyse new information, alongside that already held, in order to refine an understanding of the problem and what this might suggest should happen next. Within the confines of the problem period (problems were only on the table for a set period of time), students had to collectively appraise the situation and plan further information gathering, before the group reconvened and evaluated the situation (and possible solutions) further. The approach mimics practice insofar as it reflects the collegiate way in which practitioners need to operate, identifying their own and others' expertise and working coherently to solve a common problem (Savin-Baden, 2000; Wise, 2000).

Recognizing the anxiety that this approach might pose for students who had little or no 'expert' medical knowledge, medical educators operated as group facilitators, assisting study groups to shape their preliminary analysis of the problem and minimizing the time wasted or mistakes made during the process of investigation (Barrows, 1988). While there were useful lessons to be learned through following false lines of enquiry for a short while, and making some mistakes within the safety of the classroom, it was recognized that excess failure would lead to confusion and frustration. Students needed reasonable parameters to work within, and to sense progress, if the problem-solving case studies were to seem valuable. While students needed to be exposed to the frustration associated with learning in the real world, they also needed to feel purposeful in their investigations.

At appropriate points within the programme, medical students were assessed not only on the content knowledge accrued through investigations of problems, but upon their problem-solving skills (Barrows, 1997). While learners might not have the same volume of subject knowledge as that accrued by students studying a more traditional medical curriculum, it was argued that they had developed superior analytical skills. The skills of situation appraisal, information management and evaluation of a case were considered transferable and likely to equip students well for the varied clinical situations that would arise in the practice element of their course.

PROBLEM-BASED LEARNING COMPONENTS

Problem-based learning involves several components, which vary slightly within nursing programmes. All PBL learning, however, incorporates an educational philosophy, a framework for your learning, support and a problem-solving process. If you are reading this book in association with a programme of studies, it will be useful to compare the points made here with the explanation of PBL employed within your college. Examine how the approach is described within your programme. In this way you will be able to make accurate use of the guidance offered here, while acknowledging the assumptions that shape your course.

Educational philosophy

Problem-based learning is strongly associated with the educational values summarized in Box 2.1.

Box 2.1   Educational values and problem-based learning

1. Learning should exercise inductive and deductive processes. That is, you should gather information in order to create theories or hypotheses about the situation, and then use these to see whether these adequately explain or resolve the situation. Practitioners constantly mix and match inductive and deductive learning as part of practice development. In this way learning becomes much less superficial (Biggs, 1988).
2. You should learn within a small study group. Learning involves emotional work, notably managing anxiety. Working within a small group, you are assisted not only to manage this, but to share the responsibilities for problem-solving. The process of collaboration and challenge within the group is believed to be educationally beneficial.

3. Learning requires critical thought. To this end, educators select what free information they give to you at the outset and set questions that are designed to prompt the group to think critically. 'Trigger questions' might be used to focus your attention on specific dimensions of a situation.

4. Learning is metacognitive. Study groups are assisted by their facilitator to understand the process used to solve a problem. In many instances, you are assisted to understand your feelings and confusions *en route*.

5. Learning should encourage imagination and lateral thinking. There are often different ways to solve a problem and different sources of information or advice that could prove helpful. The process of inquiry is therefore often flexible – and you are encouraged to explore different avenues of inquiry.

6. Learning should be purposeful. It should end with a conclusion, preferably a solution to the problem. Facilitators will help your group manage inquiries so relevant goals are achieved.

7. Learning does, however, involve the construction of meanings and explanations. Within the practice world there are often no *right* answers, only better solutions. Patients and nurses often negotiate the definition of a situation and construct a plan of action that seems meaningful to both parties. Work within a study group helps you to develop the ability to construct meanings from complex or incomplete information.

While learning is seen as a group venture, each of you will retain responsibility within this. You may take it in turn to act as the chair or convenor of the study group. Other members accept responsibility for gathering particular data or suggesting possible questions and answers relevant as the problem analysis continues. All members of the group are required to challenge new information and to contribute to the debate on how, where and whether this fits into the developing analysis. With the PBL approach it is acknowledged that different group members bring different strengths and experience to the problem. Not all members can contribute in exactly the same way, or always to the same extent.

Framework for learning

Problem-based learning is also founded upon a framework, which describes how the syllabus of learning for your course and practice requirements are brought together. Nursing care scenarios are drawn from actual episodes of clinical practice, which are relevant to your current module of learning. These may be presented in a variety of formats, as patient case notes, as video clips, passages of dialogue on an audio tape or perhaps a flow chart describing the patient's experience of care in recent weeks (Barrows, 1986). What is important about such case material is that it seems authentic to real-life practice as you have observed it. With this in mind, tutors frequently include quotations from real patients and locate the case within a familiar location (e.g. an acute admissions ward). The case material is designed to provide enough intriguing points to suggest that this is worthy of your investigation. It must suggest that you and your colleagues have a role to play within the situation. It may be very brief indeed (with further information fed in later), or it may consist of an array of resources attached to a short story line (see Figure 2.1). With the case material will come tutor-prepared notes, which indicate the nature of the challenge associated with this situation. At the start of your course you may discover that case material is quite extensive, and that there are detailed guidance notes to help you begin your investigation. Later within the course the volume of material available to prompt your lines of inquiry will reduce. You will be left to interpret the situation much more independently!

The purpose of materials such as these is to help you focus your investigation upon a typical situation that is relevant to the sort of nursing work that you are, or will later, be engaged upon. The example in Figure 2.1, for instance, stems from a programme in mental health practice and focuses upon health assessment. Gary's redundancy, his position as a married man and his own self-help efforts to combat despair (sketching and drinking) are all likely to be relevant in an understanding of his

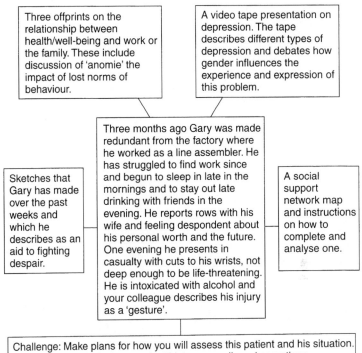

Three offprints on the relationship between health/well-being and work or the family. These include discussion of 'anomie' the impact of lost norms of behaviour.

A video tape presentation on depression. The tape describes different types of depression and debates how gender influences the experience and expression of this problem.

Three months ago Gary was made redundant from the factory where he worked as a line assembler. He has struggled to find work since and begun to sleep in late in the mornings and to stay out late drinking with friends in the evening. He reports rows with his wife and feeling despondent about his personal worth and the future. One evening he presents in casualty with cuts to his wrists, not deep enough to be life-threatening. He is intoxicated with alcohol and your colleague describes his injury as a 'gesture'.

Sketches that Gary has made over the past weeks and which he describes as an aid to fighting despair.

A social support network map and instructions on how to complete and analyse one.

Challenge: Make plans for how you will assess this patient and his situation. Ensure that this includes a patient history as well as observations.

Figure 2.1   A problem situation

situation. In this case the tutors have offered a social support network map, a device that *could* be used to assess the volume and quality of support relationships available to this patient (Price, B., 2000b).

In the event that you are planning problem-based learning as part of professional development, rather than as part of an educational programme, your own frameworks will be drawn from personal experience. They may be rather more complicated than those offered as a course presentation. Many patients have multiple problems, a complex personal and health history and have already received certain treatments or care, some of which may have failed. In order to avoid confusing yourself by the complexity of this, it will be necessary to distil the problem in one or other way. This may be done by writing down what you currently understand to be the five most important aspects of the patient's situation, or by agreeing with colleagues to focus upon a particular aspect of the patient's care. Deciding, for instance, to focus upon patient assessment, patient education, psychological support, risk management or discharge planning serves to help you shape the nature of your problem and its subsequent analysis. Williams (2001) describes this as a key skill for self-directed learning. You need to ascertain what you want to learn, and in which area this will be centred. The investigation that is to be conducted needs to have manageable parameters and this is in part determined by the first description of the situation and what you wish to discover or do about it. Box 2.2 describes the useful steps that can be completed to assist you with this.

Box 2.2   Selecting a problem for analysis

1. Identify a practice experience that did not seem to run as smoothly or as successfully as you would have wished. So much the better if it seemed to exemplify a recurrent problem in a particular aspect of your work.
2. Now distil the situation, describing what you thought were the five most important things about this situation. Try to produce a pen picture of the patient and the situation that he or she was in.
3. Identify up to five different resources, sources of additional information about the situation that were readily to hand and which you sense informed your understanding of the problem in some way. For example, this could include information from a relative, or a set of laboratory results or perhaps an extract from a textbook that you had read on the medical condition that the patient suffered from.
4. Now specify what challenge you wish to set yourself and colleagues with regard to this situation. Challenges should be of interest to all the study group members, so it is important to negotiate these. Avoid allocating yourself too many challenges in the first instance. Better to tackle a few successfully than to run out of steam tackling many.

5. Allocate yourself a reasonable project investigation time frame. Within educational programmes this is typically set within module parameters and may last one or two weeks of study. If you are investigating part-time it is usually wise to set your time parameters as one or two months. This allows scope for investigation, but it does not run on too long, risking fatigue for the group.

The second part of the framework for learning is the study or tutorial group itself. Groups may be convened for particular modules or projects, or may extend within programmes of study over a year or more. The dynamics of the study group will be pivotal to your enjoyment and success in learning (Rono, 1997; Holen, 2000; DeGrave *et al.*, 2001). It is important that all group members commit to the ethos of problem-based learning (i.e. honest inquiry, equal commitment and acknowledgement that what does not seem useful in the resolution of the problem may still represent learning of value). Problem-based learning tutorial groups may be set by tutors within college, or convened among like-minded colleagues beyond a course. PBL theorists have emphasized that the group members are not necessarily expert in any field. Indeed, they usually share a common ignorance about aspects of practice and set off together to develop expertize through their collective learning (Solomon and Crowe, 2001). No roles are predetermined within the group, but it is often agreed that all group members will act as information gatherers and data evaluators. That is, that each of you within the group will agree to, or be asked to gather particular information, which the group will then collectively evaluate at the next meeting.

In practice, it is useful for your PBL study groups to conduct two exercises before embarking upon your first investigation. The first of these consists of agreeing the etiquette of meetings, and the principles of group communication. If you are embarking upon problem-based learning for the first time it is natural to feel apprehensive about what group work will involve and feel like (Adejumo and Brysiewicz, 1998). You may be quiet and thoughtful, or extrovert and impulsive in terms of communication style, so it is helpful to agree some conventions before work begins (see Box 2.3).

Box 2.3   Study group etiquette

1. The chair of the group will rotate, as will the role of group secretary. Rotation will occur after each investigative project is completed. The chair shall be responsible (with the help of the facilitator) for summing up the current status of the investigation, welcoming contributions from the group, summarizing what has been learned, and what needs now to be investigated at each meeting. The secretary shall make notes on the meeting, using the headings, 'facts', 'learning issues', 'new inquiries' and responsibility for particular lines of inquiry.
2. Meetings will be scheduled in advance and group members will notify the secretary of any problems associated with attendance.
3. The investigative effort will be shared. The group will ensure that all group members either individually or working with colleagues investigate at least one aspect of the problem, gathering relevant information and providing a first summary of what they understand this to contribute to the problem analysis.
4. Group colleagues will listen to the report of information gathering and first summary of what this signifies without interruption. Thereafter, group members will be invited to ask questions and make suggestions concerning the new information.
5. Discussion will be constructive. New information, rather than the group colleagues, will be evaluated as part of the ongoing problem analysis.
6. The group will arrange periodic summaries of the problem analysis for consideration by the group facilitator. These will be accompanied by questions or ideas associated with how to develop the analysis further. The facilitator will not be asked to provide neat or short-cut solutions, but his or her guidance will be respected when a 'blind alley' or impasse is encountered.

Problem-based learning is in many regards more active and taxing than traditional learning where you simply write down notes from lectures or other forms of presentation (Price, B., 1998a; Gibbon, 2000). It does, however, offer much more reward. It can be extremely exciting to become an investigator or study group chair, precisely because you develop skills that will assist you in other aspects of your work. Students report feeling a 'buzz' when their investigations are going well, and a sense of achievement when they overcome an investigative problem. It is, however, important that each of your group members feels respected, and that everyone understands their responsibility to be adequately engaged in the current investigation.

The second exercise consists of inviting your colleagues to get to know one another. While much of what study group members think about nursing will unfold through problem investigations, it is often useful to gain a first summary of members' hopes, aspirations, fears and possible type of contributions at the start of the group. One simple strategy to achieve this is to ask group members to imagine that they are going on a quest. The group will form a 'fellowship', much as is described within Tolkein's popular fantasy fiction, *Lord of the Rings*. As in any heroic quest group members naturally have hopes (everyone is invited to state one or two of these), which may relate to the project ahead and/or the process of learning associated with this. Group members also have fears or concerns, so invite csolleagues to state one or two of these. Rehearsing these fears now will alert your group facilitator to concerns that might be tackled through his or her help later on. Finally, each group member is invited to characterize him or herself in terms of a contribution that *might* be useful within the group during forthcoming weeks. Contributions might be quite specific (for example, experience of conducting literature searches) or it may be rather more prosaic (for example, a sense of humour, or a comfortable way with others, encouraging them to speak their piece).

STUDENT SUPPORT

Beyond the mutual support of study group colleagues and any investigative materials supplied, or on offer through a library, a study group facilitator and a number of consultants/experts or advisers to whom you might turn will provide additional help. The terminology used to describe subject experts vary from programme to programme. However, in association with most investigations there are one or more practitioners who have specialist knowledge of relevant subjects, have conducted research within the field or who have particular expertise within an investigative process (e.g. exploring ethical issues). Such consultants are often clinical nurse specialists, subject advisers, project researchers, and field workers, although you should not assume that they will necessarily all work within nursing. We can divide such consultants into two groups as follows:

Education-briefed advisers

Consultants or advisers who are education briefed are not only authoritative within their own subject field but they have received briefing on the problem-based learning approach and the case study situations being explored by you and your colleagues. They appreciate the focus of your investigations and may have given additional thought to their own practice experience in dealing with just these issues. This is not to suggest, however, that education-briefed advisers stand ready to provide you with fast track or instant answers to the problems that you investigate. Instead, they are likely to provide answers with reflections that demonstrate insight into the inquiry process that you are undertaking. Within some college programmes there may be several education-briefed consultants or mentors who undertake to welcome your inquiries and who develop considerable experience in answering questions and assisting you to appreciate the scope or dimensions of a problem.

Subject-informed advisers

Other subject experts, consultants or advisers express a willingness to assist you with your studies but have not received briefing or training in problem-based learning techniques. Subject-informed consultants might therefore provide you with information, but do not have special expertise in helping you to shape your questions or evaluate the information accruing from discussion.

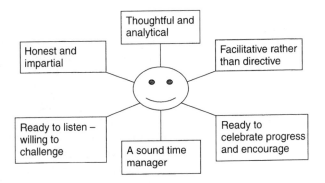

Figure 2.2   Personal qualities of the study group facilitator

Because of the significant cost in preparing staff to assist with problem-based learning programmes or initiatives, it is likely that subject-informed consultants will outnumber those who are education briefed.

The main support to your study group, however, is provided by a study group facilitator (Neville, 1999; Murray and Savin-Baden, 2000). If this role is fulfilled by a college tutor, he or she will normally have been trained in group facilitation skills, be familiar with the problem-based learning approach and is likely to have been engaged in writing or updating some of the case study materials that you investigate. If you are conducting your problem-based learning studies independent of a programme or course, it will be important to identify a study group facilitator from among your more experienced colleagues. Individuals with experience of student support within practice areas, those who have conducted research or practice projects of their own and those who express a fascination with learning to practical ends are likely to make better group facilitators under these circumstances. It will be important to select a facilitator, however, who has a number of other more personal qualities (see Figure 2.2).

There has been extensive debate concerning whether a study group facilitator should be a subject expert (e.g. De Volder, 1982; Moust and Schmidt, 1992; Zeitz and Paul, 1993). Those that are expert within a subject field might be tempted to 'teach' rather than facilitate your investigation. However comforting that might seem to you and your colleagues, it is unlikely to help you develop the inquisitive skills that will serve you well within health care. Study group facilitators who are not expert, and may even be a peer (i.e. ignorant of much of the subject, but keen to assist you in your discoveries) may prolong your investigations, simply because they are less sure when the group is exploring a blind alley.

Neville (1999) provides an extensive review of the role of the problem-based learning tutor (or study group facilitator). He draws upon the work of Knowles (1975) discussing the functions that a learning facilitator is involved in (see Box 2.4). Within the context of problem-based learning, however, study group facilitators focus their work in two ways: upon guiding the work of the group, and promoting interaction (Wilkerson, 1992).

Box 2.4   Tutor roles in facilitated learning

1. Climate creation (helping you to become acquainted and to value the purpose of the group).
2. Planning facilitation (helping your group create plans of action).
3. Designing learning needs (helping your group decide what you need to investigate successfully).
4. Setting goals (either those required within a syllabus or assisting you to set your own beyond that).
5. Designing a learning strategy (helping you to consider the different ways in which you could proceed, setting schedules and time frames).
6. Engaging in learning activities (deciding upon a role and level of intervention, what will be told and questioned, what will be prompted or supported).
7. Evaluating learning outcomes (helping your group to audit your progress).

Source: Adapted from Knowles (1975)

Your study group facilitator will use a number of skills to help you 'shape your investigation'. At the outset this will include conducting an appreciation of the task ahead of you. It is important to clarify what you believe the challenge consists of. Misinterpreting this at the outset can lead to wasted time and unpromising results. Skilful study group facilitators find a balance between listening to you and talking about the project or your group work to date. When your facilitator does talk, you may discover that he or she is using a number of techniques to facilitate your learning (see Figure 2.3).

Facilitators use probing (a series of questions) to understand what you currently think, whether you all agree on a subject and to help illustrate lines of inquiry (MacHaffie, 1988). For example, if you are tackling a project on breast-feeding which requires you to consider why women elect not to breast-feed and then to identify the merits of health education about this, the facilitator might probe what each of you believe about breast-feeding. The purpose of this is not to cause division within the group itself, but to encourage you to rehearse the possible motives that an individual may have for electing to breast- or bottle-feed a baby. By discovering your own attitudes and beliefs you will not only understand how you think or feel, but quite possibly uncover important material that needs investigation as part of your work on health education in this context! To be on the receiving end of probing questions can seem uncomfortable, especially if you do not understand, or trust the motives of the questioner. It is important therefore to think critically about what the probe questions might reveal to you. In what ways might the probes suggest possible lines of inquiry or ways of thinking about the problem that you may have missed? While your facilitator may genuinely want to understand what you think (meeting his or her own needs), there is usually something that you can glean from this. We shall be returning to different styles of questioning

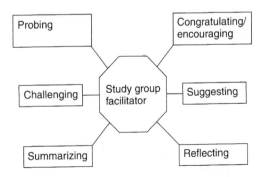

Figure 2.3 Facilitation of your learning

in subsequent chapters, particularly when we discuss the collection of data (Chapter 4) and the evaluation of information (Chapter 5).

At other times, study group facilitators challenge your thinking – they play 'devil's advocate' (MacDougall and Baum, 1997). When first used this can seem quite startling. Not only does it make you question your own progress, your current perspective or even your own confidence, but it forces you to reconsider just what role the facilitator is playing. A traditional teacher often acts as an information giver, a fact provider, so to be questioned by such an authoritative figure might suggest that he or she really does not know what is best or right. If the facilitator needs to challenge you, perhaps he or she does not know the answer? Alternatively, the facilitator may seem prejudiced or opinionated, arguing from an ideological basis about what *should* be. Sound educational challenge is used by a facilitator, however, when it seems possible that you have foreclosed an argument, deciding that something is right or clear before, in fact, all the possibilities have been considered. A challenge might be used when you appear complacent, or when the facilitator senses that group members are moving off in different directions. Paradoxically a challenge sometimes prompts group members to drop their differences and to focus together upon what the facilitator is posing. Study group facilitators are usually experienced in the use of challenge, although they do not use this technique lightly. As time progresses, you will usually be encouraged to challenge others yourself. Challenge is a normal part of problem-solving.

Facilitators also congratulate and encourage. There will be times in projects where you deserve to be congratulated upon progress, the way in which you have tackled a part of the investigation. Really effective congratulations and encouragement are delivered in two parts. The first describes what has gone well while the second explains why this was praiseworthy. If you receive congratulations from your facilitator, look for both parts. It is in the second part of the message that you will learn most from the experience of being patted on the back. Congratulation is often offered when you have completed a stage or section of an investigation. At such times the facilitator will normally take stock of what you have now achieved and why this stage was important to complete as part of the larger project. When the facilitator does this, he or she is 'summarizing' – helping you to audit trail what you have already done and what (by implication) may yet need to be achieved.

You may be surprised to discover that study group facilitators suggest things, possible lines of inquiry, alternative interpretations, additional questions, or possible explanations of phenomena in a very measured way. Facilitators are encouraged to avoid directing or controlling the problem analysis. Within the constraints of time it is more important for you to inquire, rather than for you to follow the instructions of the group facilitator. Study group facilitators take time to learn where best, how much and how often to contribute ideas into the group. Like good research supervisors they try to help you mine useful information and to avoid unduly constraining your options. There may, however, come times when the group is struggling, or travelling along an unhelpful path, and the facilitator suggests one or two ideas. These are often seeds to help you kick start your inquiry or to gently warn you that the line of inquiry is drying up.

Slightly less directive than suggestions is reflection. Successful study group facilitators will sometimes 'muse aloud' about a current debate that you are having. Consider, for example, an investigation where you are exploring the ethical dimensions of clinical decisions. Your reading has alerted you to the fact that ethical decisions might be based upon ethical principles (deontological) or upon anticipated consequences of action or inaction (teleological) (Burckhardt, 2002). You may act upon the principle of beneficence, for instance, or upon a review of what might happen to this patient if you do not proceed in a particular way. Within ethics there is so often no clear-cut solution, but it is useful to 'massage the arguments'. A facilitator pauses at this moment to illustrate the pros and cons of different perspectives. He or she is role modelling a reasoning process and one that might assist you with the current, or a later problem.

Reflection is sometimes used by facilitators to help you resolve differences of opinion within the group. Periodically, problem-based learning investigations throw up issues which help you to realize what you are passionate about and what you understand to be sound/correct/moral or effective nursing practice (see Chapter 1). At these points, your facilitator may 'time out' the investigation briefly and encourage group members to pause and examine their own values and beliefs. Such a facilitated reflection may be offered one to one and in private, or as part of a small group discussion. The important point here is that reflection can assist you with a problem analysis or a study group process!

PROBLEM-SOLVING PROCESS

The final component of problem-based learning is the problem-solving process. Since PBL approaches were first used within health care curricula, problem-solving processes have been refined and modified (Glen and Wilkie, 2000). In part, the problem-solving process is a function of the PBL philosophy, partly a function of the case study design, partly a product of the study group dynamic and is frequently associated with the constraints of time or other resources. This said, a number of things could be said about the process with confidence. These include the following:

1. Problem analysis moves from coarse analysis to refined analysis. That is, we often think of problems in simplistic terms at first and as we unpack them we discover they are multi-faceted and more complex. We need to ask more discrete or specific questions and to understand aspects of behaviour or practice in a more measured way.
2. As a result of moving towards a more refined analysis, problems become bigger or more complex before they are resolved. Its really rather like blowing up a balloon that you hope won't explode in your face. You need to expand the problem analysis to the optimum point and then understand when to tie things off, and appreciate it for what it is.
3. Problem-solving involves a series of cycles, that start with first appraisal of the problem, what it consists of, what the challenge(s) are and what you already know about this. After this, the group identify what they do not understand, what they do not know, and surmise where such information might be found out. The group now enters a data-gathering phase, before reconvening to discuss what has been gleaned from other sources and to ascertain what this now tells us about the problem. Within some projects (time permitting), you may undertake a number of cycles, data gathering–data analysing–action planning in order to reach a point where you think you understand the problem, possible solutions and what constitutes the most artful, safe or effective response. At this level, problem-based learning has much in common with action research (Coghlan and Casey, 2001).

| **Working solutions** |
| Tentative accounts of 'what is going on' and what now may need to be done. |

Learning issues		**New inquiries**
That which you do not know but need to understand or investigate in some way. That which still seems contentious or controversial.		What you will now source, where you will now look to resolve learning issues.

| **Facts** |
| Information you understand to be corroborated and sound. This is information that underpins all other parts of your investigation. |

Figure 2.4   Recording the problem investigation

Because PBL investigations can generate a massive amount of different information and you must elect what such information means in the context of the problem, it is helpful to use a record system that helps you keep track of the problem trail (see Figure 2.4). This consists of sheets of paper (I recommend A3 size) or computer records that describe the problem in terms of facts, learning issues, new inquiries and 'working solutions'.

As a group you will need to agree when information can be placed within the 'fact compartment' of your record. For information to constitute a fact you will need to feel that you have critically examined it, that it is supported by evidence from other sources (it seems corroborated in some manner), and that it is manifestly relevant to the nature of the challenge before you. It's very easy to admit information as fact too quickly and then to discover that you cannot agree on the focus of the problem or possible solutions. To return to our balloon analogy above, you need to consider how much air you blow into the balloon. Too much hot air is likely to burst the balloon.

Learning issues refers to the bag of information, debates, ideas and arguments that continue to be unresolved within your analysis to date. As investigations develop you are likely to accumulate learning issues and it will be necessary periodically to consider whether some or all of these remain relevant to the investigation in hand. Sometimes there will be a need to resolve a difference of perspective, to accept one perspective as more authoritative than another or to accept that some concepts or ideas are simply more helpful on this occasion. By keeping a record of what has been left on the table in any problem analysis you will be able to sense when this has grown large and it is now imperative to delay further data gathering and to conclude some analysis work.

New inquiries refers to the group's plan of action regarding where they think new and valuable information may be found, or where expertize might be sought to help you resolve a learning issue. New inquiries can be used to detail just who will gather new information, what form of data gathering that will take (e.g. a trip to the library, interviewing others) and what the focus of inquiry will be. This is an important part of the investigative process because if sources and focus of inquiry are not carefully planned, information may be poor or incomplete.

Significantly in Figure 2.4 learning issues and new inquiries rest upon facts and support 'working solutions'. Students often wonder how a problem solution is evolved, and may even imagine that it just springs forth from the analysis (Price, 1998a). In reality, solutions are often proposed and then abandoned. The group 'tries out solutions' to see if they fit with the nature of the challenge, the problem circumstances, and whether they are adequately supported by facts, investigations and inquiries. Towards the end of an investigation, therefore, groups tend to generate tentative solutions. The volume of new information and lines of inquiry start to fall away and the group concentrates rather more on analysis and inquiries designed to test the veracity of their tentative solutions. Group facilitators have a key role in helping you realize when it is feasible to start testing possible solutions. Facilitators help you examine the problem analysis to see whether it seems structurally sound.

CONCLUSION

While problem-based learning has its origins within medical schools, it has become an effective and widely disseminated educational approach across health care. Within nursing, PBL curricula are now common. Its potential as an approach to professional update learning and/or practice development has yet to be fully explored. This is in part because problem-based learning has relied heavily upon the design of case study materials and upon the expertize of study group facilitators who help learners to manage the size and direction of the investigations. For PBL to succeed beyond the college curriculum it will be important for study groups to identify a skilful group facilitator and to set realistic goals and challenges regarding the problems to be solved.

What characterizes the PBL approach to inquiry is the exploration of problems before theory has been comprehensively taught. This mimics the inductive–deductive investigations familiar in clinical practice and fosters the development of group working skills, which are important within health care. PBL requires you to examine not only what the problem is and which solutions might be useful, but the processes by which the solutions have been arrived at. Successful problem-based learning therefore helps you to develop metacognitive skills and an understanding of how to analyse practice situations.

While it is possible to conduct group work learning using other approaches, problem-based learning works with a distinctive philosophy that you will need to understand and respect. Respecting this philosophy will mean that you gain the most from working with a study group facilitator, other colleagues within the study group and the mentors or consultants who might inform your study. Problem-based learning involves a journey, using particular case study materials and a series of stages which identify the problem, and refine your analysis of this, before enabling you to move towards tentative solutions.

Having now read this chapter it is useful to reflect, how does this approach to learning seem to you? Clearly, it demands personal organization and commitment to group work. It is an inherently active form of study, with significant rewards. While investigations may involve periods of confusion and anxiety, they also contain discoveries that are intensely satisfying and motivating. When you pause to consider what you learn from a course that is of lasting value, you may conclude that it is not the facts, theories or science, but the techniques by which you can continue to learn and solve problems of your own.

3 ENQUIRY-BASED LEARNING

If problem-based learning has a clear historical root within medical education, enquiry-based learning (EBL) has a more confused lineage. This is partly because EBL has sometimes been seen as a variant on problem-based learning, expressing a different philosophy (that is, practice cannot always result in cure or resolution of problems, but it still requires exploration of different options and meanings). It is also partly because some authors have preferred to use 'EBL' to 'PBL' as a semantic representation of that which is most central within small group study. Such authors reflect that inquiry is at the heart of such learning, and some of them then debate whether it should be termed enquiry- or inquiry-based learning (Inouye and Flannelly, 1998). Like many other education and nursing innovations, the longer a new approach has been exposed to interpretation and the wider it has spread (geographically and through disciplines), the more attenuated the theory often becomes. At one level this seems disappointing because it could appear to dilute the central tenets of the strategy. At another level, however, variation may reflect the needs of local learning, the cultural context of education. Just how you view such matters depends on whether you see variation as opportunity, or confusion, making it more difficult to understand what you are about to become engaged with.

In this volume, then, I will define enquiry-based learning in a particular way and consistently refer to EBL rather than IBL. My definition of EBL is based upon distinctions that I argue may be drawn with problem-based learning and upon the notion that enquiry-based learning has a significant role to play within professional update and practice development (e.g. Price and Price, 2000; Price, B., 2001a). Experience of working with nurses and others operating within practice settings suggests to me that the EBL vehicle offers an exciting opportunity to link professional update learning to practice development. Using the EBL approach you might study far more actively than you would otherwise do so through study days or conferences. You will develop the sort of inquisitive, transferable and co-operative skills so important to practice development. You will also make a meaningful contribution to the quality of local health care services through projects conducted with other professionals. I suggest that, subject to adequate support and supervision, such enquiry-based learning represents not just a viable professional update option within hospitals and elsewhere, but one which pays considerable dividends to employers as well as yourself.

DISTINCTIONS BETWEEN ENQUIRY- AND PROBLEM-BASED LEARNING

At the outset, it is important to point out that both problem- and enquiry-based learning approaches share a number of philosophical premises first introduced in Box 2.1. Simply put, these are that you have a great deal to gain from active study that involves you in inductive and deductive thinking and which requires that you work closely with others, within small study groups, to make sense of the practice environment and the challenges that exist there. Enquiry-based learning is equally concerned with learning that is relevant to the practice situation, and which develops the sorts of transferable skills that have greatest value to practitioners. Accordingly, enquiry-based learning is not shaped by topics or traditional divisions of learning, but by means of inquiry, and the ethos of discovering information. You need to 'theorize in practice', creating accounts of what is happening and then examining whether these assist you with your professional work (Price, 1998a).

Enquiry-based learning also shares the precepts that attend problem-based learning. That is, it is accepted that investigations work best when they are facilitated and when there is a definable process of information gathering and information analysis, through the study group. Group projects, conducted without the aid of supervision or facilitation, are likely to founder, either because they do not have strategy and clear direction or because the group attempt projects that are too large, or too vague to sustain motivation. Enquiry-based learning shares the PBL focus upon discussion, challenge and support within the study group. It supports the notion that projects must work to a purpose and that these are necessarily resource-limited.

Beyond this, however, there are some subtle distinctions that are important for those of you who read this textbook after you have completed programmes of education and those who are reading it alongside study on a PBL or traditional nursing syllabus.

THE AIM OF ENQUIRY-BASED LEARNING

While the aim of problem-based learning has been to identify and evaluate solutions to a health care practice problem, the purpose of enquiry-based learning is to understand the nature of health care practice more sensitively. I accept the argument that there are aspects of practice which are not open to reso-lution yet which require the practitioner to develop principles of practice that might be of assistance in the future. Health care work sometimes requires that the patient and practitioner explore the significance or meaning of situations and need to discover a working arrangement that helps the patient to cope with new circumstances. Just as medicine cannot always cure all diseases or rectify physical or mental health faults, so nursing cannot always relieve the patient of responsibility to cope with change. Nurses have to think in pragmatic ways, assisting patients to create accounts of their circumstances, and best fit responses that enable them to live as independently, and as confidently as possible (Price, 1998b). In this sense, nurses neither provide a solution to the problem, nor direct the patient to one that could simply be replicated from elsewhere. Instead, the nurse facilitates new ways of living, and assists the patient to learn through health or illness experiences (Peplau, 1994).

Beyond this philosophical point about the orientation of some aspects of nursing care it is arguable that nurses engage in a number of practice approaches which are used with different patients and many circumstances over time. Chapter 1 acknow-ledges the different ways in which practitioners understand the purpose of care. There is therefore a case to be made for understanding this work much more deeply. Not only might this result in more sensitive expression of nursing care, but it might also illuminate the circumstances under which approaches need

Table 3.1 Nursing approaches and enquiry-based learning

Practice context	Care approach	Rationale of interest
Altered body image rehabilitation	Helping patients accommodate or adjust body image	Should body image change be seen as something to resist or resolve, or something that should be adapted to?
Patient history taking	Emphasis upon understanding disease (signs or events) or upon understanding illness (experiences and symptoms)	There is finite time to take a patient history but this often 'opens' the care relationship. How we approach this influences how patients see us and understand our role

particular attention or adjustment. In Table 3.1 I illustrate these points with reference to two sample nursing approaches.

In these examples there is an emphasis upon practice contexts that extend beyond individual patients and events. Altered body rehabilitation continues with new patients, when previous patients have gone home. Patient history taking recurs day in day out with a sequence of patients and there is the prospect that we might learn something from this context, even if the patients and problems change (Price and Price, 2000). The purpose of enquiry-based learning is therefore to inform practice and fuel practice development. There may be scant time to use problem analysis to tackle an individual patient's problems, and merit in learning principles of sound practice that could inform different situations.

The second important point concerns the nature of care approaches. Notice how these refer to the style, assumptions or ways of approaching practice. These may reflect a personal philosophy of nursing care, a corporate protocol or an assessment of what the nurse understands the public expects. They are not necessarily problems, but they are issues that require the nurse to take a stance, or proceed in particular ways as situations arise. In the first example, two possible care approaches are identified. The first frames altered body image as a problem, a blemish or shortfall, associated with illness, trauma or treatment that the patient will probably want rectified. This approach assumes that the patient understands body image change in cathexis terms (that is, as a challenge to his or her satisfaction with body function or appearance). The second approach frames altered body image as a change process, albeit one that is accelerated within illness or injury. Within this care approach the role of the nurse is perceived to focus upon helping patients accommodate change. Just as people adapt to changes in physical appearance associated with ageing, so they may be assisted to adapt to more abrupt changes. Because patients adopt different attitudes regarding this, and nurses approach rehabilitation practice with different orientations about what is to be done, the practice deserves additional scrutiny in case colleagues might learn something from the analysis (e.g. Newell, 1999).

A similar, and quite fundamental challenge is associated with how nurses approach patient history taking. Textbooks may emphasize one or other approach, some data more than others, but the nurse is left to cope with arranging history taking in different contexts (Morton, 1989). It is possible to take different nursing approaches to history taking, one of which pays greater attention to illness as experience and meaning, and one of which places greater emphasis upon empirical data and risk management. In practice, nurses combine questions from both approaches, and then may, or may not feel satisfied with the sort of data that they record, or the subsequent relationship they establish with the patient.

Enquiry-based projects prepared in these contexts may be devised to answer a number of questions. These include the following:

- Why do we practise in this way?
- Under what conditions or circumstances, do our approaches change?
- Are there situations when we should rethink our approaches?
- Where we operate differently as practitioners, should we consider consolidating nursing approaches? If so, to what purpose?
- How do others see our nursing approaches – are there advantages/disadvantages, challenges or opportunities here?

These questions are rather different from those formulated in problem-based learning, where the emphasis is sometimes upon one patient or situation, and where there is an opening assumption that some form of coherent solution might be arrived at. What characterizes questions formed within enquiry-based learning is that they are focused upon a journey – a discovery that will not necessarily render a discrete answer, but which may sensitize the nurse to practice, and assist her to explain what she is attempting or assist others with similar challenges. Enquiry-based learning therefore has the purpose of making implicit reasoning and tacit knowledge explicit (see Eraut, 1990, for further account of tacit knowledge). Its purpose is to help colleagues learn through investigation, unpacking that which previously may have been described as intuitive or hidden. Where common agreement is reached upon practices, then it may include recommendation of worthwhile or best practice to others.

ENQUIRY-BASED LEARNING AND PROJECT TIME

Because EBL study groups are working towards a greater understanding of practice, rather than a problem solution, it is more difficult for you to sense when to close a project and to move on to other matters. Project time is, however, an important consideration in enquiry-based learning, precisely because to over-extend an investigation may be to disillusion or confuse the study group, while to confine an investigation to too little project time may be to frustrate aspirations. In EBL therefore it is important to set realistic project time frames that are likely to facilitate significant learning, but which will not exhaust you. Table 3.2 indicates some of the ways in which an EBL project can be successfully time-framed.

Within enquiry-based learning the study group facilitator, consultee/sponsor or project advisers play a prominent time manager role. Skilful group facilitators help your group to establish a maximum project time, but within this they search for an appropriate time to suggest that significant learning has been achieved and the project has reached either a resting place (where it can be picked up on another date) or closure. Assuming that your group may wish to embark on new projects, and to work together in the future, it is often just as important to know

Table 3.2   Time-framing EBL studies

Time frame control	Source	Rationale
Group facilitator	Inside group	A carefully selected group facilitator explores your interests and expectations with you. She monitors the project, its direction and progress, seeking the right moment for a project to close on a satisfying note
Consultee or sponsor	Outside group	Some EBL projects are sponsored and include a pre-set project time frame
Project scope external advisers	Outside group	Like other health care projects there is usually a need to 'scope the project'. That is, the group must decide how many and which goals will be pursued within a finite time. Experts on different health issues may advise upon this

when to leave a project, because its prolongation would damage morale. Experienced sponsors or consultees, perhaps a consultant nurse, clinical nurse specialist or other service manager, offer project time frames that are some 10–20 per cent more generous in terms of time than they believe it may take to achieve a new direction or a clearer approach to practice. This allows for the exploration of blind alleys, the expression of individual learning needs within the group, and the chance for you to develop some interpersonal and transferable skills. Project commissioning remains a skilful business, and there may come moments when the consultee or sponsor needs to compare notes with the group facilitator in order to decide whether to foreclose on a project or suggest an extension of time. External advisers are often able to recommend time frames, using their knowledge of research within a particular field. Either way, at the outset, it is important to think of time management as an important part of your investigation.

ENQUIRY-BASED LEARNING SUPPORT

If you are studying a PBL approach course syllabus the arrangements for the support of your study group are largely pre-set. Different academic and clinical staff are inducted into support roles (Drummond-Young, 1998). The nature of what help the facilitator is meant to provide is in large part shaped by the curriculum and the sort of case studies and trigger questions that are asked of you. Within enquiry-based learning, study group support relies upon a study group facilitator to do rather more (see Figure 3.1).

Some of the earliest support work is associated with scoping the project and finding a project focus. Scoping refers to agreeing the extent of the project, how many goals will be pursued and over what period of time. It involves helping your group to establish to what extent you will investigate aspects of practice. This usually means a compromise if the project is to retain the interest of all group members, but to also remain viable within the available time frame. Before this, though, and in situations where a group of practitioners know they want to explore something concerning a subject, but they're not quite sure what, there may be a need for the facilitator to help you settle upon an acceptable focus. Take a look now at Box 3.1, which provides two accounts of just this sort of process, from the perspective of a group member, and the group facilitator.

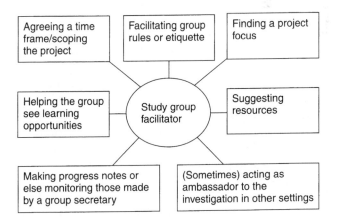

Figure 3.1 Group facilitator duties (EBL)

Box 3.1   Finding a focus

Group member (a supervisor of midwives)

While there didn't seem to be anything especially wrong with the different ways we were dealing with third stage labour, several of us were aware that midwives took very different approaches to it. We couldn't put our finger on the focus exactly, but we wanted to think about this, without unduly threatening anyone through the process. I thought, if I do this through supervision, it could feel heavy-handed.

Group facilitator

At first I thought the group were interested in how they went about assessing women's labour. It took a conversation or two to realize that this was just the context though. What they were really interested in was grasping a tougher nettle. There were different attitudes to the level of intervention that should be used in such circumstances. There were natural birth folk and what might be described as 'interventionists'. These brave midwives wanted to explore the different perspectives not because they thought they could win an argument, but because they wanted to understand where colleagues were coming from. They thought they might work better together as a result.

In a paper describing practice-based learning of this sort, Price and Price (2000) highlight the importance of a group facilitator spotting learning opportunities that help the group to clarify their focus and add something new to the investigation. A successful group facilitator is often a lateral thinker, who spots the similarities that can arise within different situations. If your group focuses upon an abstract concept (e.g. sensitive information giving), there may be many incidents and opportunities for group members to draw inferences from observations in practice. At such times it is important for the group facilitator to alert you all to the learning that may be on offer. For example, information giving to colleagues, in terms of technique *might* teach us something about information giving in other circumstances. Lessons learned about cultural communication in other contexts *might* offer something interesting in the current project context.

It may surprise you to read that sometimes the group facilitator may be called upon to be the ambassador of the project in other contexts. This arises frequently enough, however, when other stakeholders feel that they are becoming onlookers to reflections upon practice that they believe may affect them. EBL projects may either represent or suggest change to others. Change within health care practice can seem threatening, especially if this challenges traditional professional boundaries, or questions the ethics of a particular practice approach. Employers and managers may feel threatened when practice is investigated at 'grass-roots level' and without commission from their office. Such concerns become very real within health care services where there is an increasingly flattened hierarchy of leadership, and where divisions between what managers and clinicians lead on become blurred (Rippon and Monaghan, 2001). While EBL does not claim to solve problems or to provide distinctive answers about what *must* be done, there is still a need for the project to be represented fairly and constructively to others. Equally, other stakeholders (if they have not been persuaded to join the group) need to have their ideas considered. Study group facilitators are better placed than group members to represent the inquiry. This is not only because the facilitator understands the investigation in overview, but because he or she is not immediately engaged in data gathering and analysis (something that can temporarily blind the investigator to the broader picture).

CHOOSING A GROUP FACILITATOR

Assuming that you have found a group of like-minded, and multi-disciplinary inquisitive professionals with whom to form a group, you are collectively now faced with the responsibility to find and select a group facilitator. Just whom do you choose and what qualities should you seek in this colleague? Many of the qualities that make for an excellent PBL study group facilitator also apply to the EBL facilitator (see Box 3.2). He or she will need

---

Box 3.2   Qualities and background of the EBL facilitator

Personal qualities

Integrity – a person willing to be clear and consistent, honest and equitable in his or her treatment of group members.

Analytical – able to see the overview, and to sense progress, blind alleys and useful avenues.

Reflective/reflexive – able to examine ideas aloud, his/her own and yours. Can your chosen person 'think aloud' in much the same way as an advanced driver has to talk aloud thoughts and intentions during an examination?

Humour – for those moments when everyone needs to laugh at their predicament.

Positive – someone who looks for the achievements and highlights the learning.

Inquisitive and passionate about learning – whatever the outcome, this person needs to care about what you learn, and how the experience feels for you.

Professional backgrounds (one or more may prove helpful)

The clinical supervisor – experience in reflection and helping others make their own exploratory practice journey.

The researcher – experience of structuring investigations, and managing timescales and resources.

The consultant – used to working with others' agendas and helping them meet their goals.

The field expert/consultant nurse – rich provider of resources, or networker who can put group members in touch with other experts.

The project manager – worldly wise about managing the professional/corporate interface, the politician who understands the service as well as the practitioners.

---

personal qualities, but because there may have been no formal preparation for this role, save for books on PBL/EBL study, it will be important to think about people who develop parallel skills in other contexts.

It is inappropriate to suggest that one particular background is right for every EBL inquiry. On the contrary, provided that you have a clear focus for your investigation already, there is merit in choosing a group facilitator with this in mind. For example, a project that you believe will involve significant data gathering and access arrangements, within a group where you feel ready to challenge any over-zealous steering by an expert, may encourage you to approach a consultant nurse or project manager. Such individuals might offer considerable expertize in putting you in touch with others, or alerting you to research evidence already published. Alternatively, if your project is about exploring attitudes and approaches to practice, and you sense that the debate could prove emotive, it may be important to approach a consultant or clinical supervisor from another division of the hospital. You seek someone with considerable group skills, 'no axe to grind' and who will be sincerely interested in helping you develop your ideas.

Upon balance, I suggest that personal qualities are most important. Your facilitator should have good interpersonal skills and experience of working sensitively with groups in one or other setting. The facilitator needs the personal discipline to stand back and help you conduct your investigations, and the strength of mind to appreciate when it is necessary to intervene. Ask this question: were we to disagree about something as a group, would we respect this person enough to trust her or him to direct what needs to be done next?

THE ENQUIRY PROCESS

If problem-based learning can be said to develop through a process of problem formulation, problem deconstruction, solution formation and conclusion then enquiry-based learning also has a certain shape (Price, B., 2001a) (see Figure 3.2).

We have already alluded to the role of the group facilitator in helping to find an enquiry focus. In practical terms, however, we need to consider what this means. One possible approach to finding a focus for EBL study is therefore to consider whether one or more aspects of practice are of prime interest to the group (e.g. assessing, decision-making, teaching, counselling). Using a white board or large sheet of paper divided up into compartments, one for each aspect of practice, it is possible to

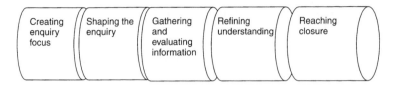

Figure 3.2   The EBL process
Source: Price, B., 2001a

state questions, interests or aims regarding each. In some projects there may be little or no interest in particular aspects. Experience of project management, however, suggests that while the group may not start their inquiries with a particular aspect, they may still detour through others at some point, precisely because discussions uncover assumptions or values that are important there.

To illustrate this focusing exercise, consider the situation of a group of nurses and other health care professionals who work with clinically obese patients. While they come from different specialities (e.g. diabetes care, peripheral vascular surgery, mental health), they share a common interest in the well-being of patients and a concern that unless obesity is tackled there may be severe consequences (Brownell, 1998). They consider the beliefs that they use in their approach to such patients and agree that obese people *should* lose weight and adjust their lifestyle so as to manage their body weight more effectively. The practitioners' role is therefore seen as promotional and instructive – encouraging patients to follow dietary and related advice. Next, they consider the knowledge that practitioners use to promote healthier lifestyles and note that there is a preponderance of knowledge about physiology and pathology, and rather less about psychology and lifestyle. They are also aware that they have few skills regarding the assessment of lifestyle, or concerning the facilitation of learning. The group facilitator queries, 'Do you think that your interest is in making health promotion more actionable with patients – are you wanting to get beyond ideas about what should happen, to understanding what you need to know or do to help make it happen for clients?' The group agree – there is gap between theory and reality, between philosophy and practice.

In most projects the process of focusing upon a practice slips quickly into shaping the enquiry. Flannelly and Inouye (1998), for instance, talk about conceptualizing the situation. To extend our example about shaping this investigation now depends upon discussing a number of concepts so that the investigators understand the nature of what they are dealing with. There may, for instance, be a discrepancy between what is considered clinically obese in terms of body mass index and what patients and practitioners agree is just being 'overweight'. The study group may need to agree what they are talking about – whether inquiries will focus upon what is involved upon helping patients achieve a clinical or a personally acceptable body weight! At this stage, differences of opinion can arise and it is important to address these before the group plan their investigations in detail (Milligan, 1999).

The process of gathering and sifting information shares much in common with the PBL practice described in Chapter 2. EBL investigators proceed through a series of rounds, gathering more information and sifting this in the light of what has already been gleaned. The practical details of such work are described in Chapters 5 and 6 of this book. There are, however, some differences between EBL and PBL with regard to evaluating the information that has been gathered. While within PBL the group consider information in terms of whether it constitutes facts that can be accepted as a given with regard to the rest of the investigation, within EBL it may be impossible for the group to agree that information is quite so solid. On the contrary, as the investigation progresses, the group may discover that a practice becomes more and more complex and that at best various pieces of information can be considered 'significant'. There is an outstanding debate to be conducted concerning how the information fits with other information, or guides thinking. For this reason, EBL often carries a greater baggage of possibly significant information and challenges the group to consider how the information fits together. Drawing upon our example once more, it may for instance be significant that adults within the western world lead a more sedentary lifestyle because of the nature of work. Office work, commuting and the computer may all contribute to a less physical style of working. It remains questionable, however, whether this is amenable to change, or whether the practitioner should concentrate upon the peripheral activities of leisure time (negative or positive).

As with PBL processes, the group moves (over time) towards a more refined understanding of the situation. In the case of EBL, understanding that attends to what is important or influential, that which could be focused upon as open to change or further study, rather than that which must be solved. The EBL process leads to a greater appreciation of where practitioners are powerful, where they have the potential to influence, and where they are yet missing important education or resources. In some regards EBL involves refining our understanding of the situation. As one student analogized it, 'You don't have a plan for logging every tree off the mountain, because you're not sure that you should. You do though know the wood from the trees and understand what is out there.'

EBL study groups need to reach a closure rather than to propose a solution. Price observes:

> In any investigation there comes a point when the group must decide whether to continue investigating or to draw conclusions about what has been discovered so far. If the investigation is EBL, an alternative question arises: do we now have enough information to help us understand the situation better and prompt new ways of working?
>
> (Price, B., 2001a, p. 51)

Price cautions against foreclosing upon an investigation where it has relied upon a few (influential) sources of information. Studies are usually more complete if a variety of sources have been tapped and different types and formats of information considered (Price, B., 2001a). The conclusion to the project might then be written up using a number of headings (see Box 3.3).

Box 3.3 EBL conclusions

Description

The group describe the practice or subject in more refined terms. Its complexity and importance are now highlighted, indicating that the group have moved beyond the 'common sense' or 'folk wisdom' understanding of it.

Goals

The goals of the investigation are restated, together with comments on what was not attainable. This enables others to appreciate the progress of the group.

Findings

While the group is unlikely to present findings in terms of facts, there is likely to be a series of issues/knowledge/ decisions/approaches which are considered to be more significant. This alerts the reader to areas of practice that might benefit from priority attention. The findings suggest which elements of practice have a major bearing upon the practice issue or inquiry subject.

Cautions

The group acknowledge a number of points about what has not been tapped, understood or debated in full.

Implications

Before suggesting why such an investigation is important to local practice.

Source: After Price (2001a)

In Chapter 11 you have an opportunity to examine a sample EBL investigation and the closure that was reached there. At this stage, however, it is important to indicate that the findings and implications do not equate with research findings. Findings may seem tentative, indicating areas of concern, foci where practice outcomes are strongly influenced. The implications do not necessarily direct the reader to what *should* now be done, but invite her or him to consider, 'What does this mean for how you practise?' Alternatively, 'What does this mean for how you think about these issues?'

CONCLUSION

We have now reached the end of an admittedly eclectic account of enquiry-based learning, and the ways in which it might be distinguished from problem-based learning. In part, the distinctions are academic in that both approaches to learning are concerned with discovery and thinking afresh about practice.

Where the distinctions become significant, however, is when I make the case that within nursing and related health care, there will remain aspects of practice that are not open to problem solving. Health care will remain interpretive, requiring the practitioner to think how *could* I behave here? What might seem more useful in this situation, not because it solves a problem *per se*, but because it is more artistic, more sensitive or likely to help us work together better in the future? As we shall see within the next chapter, there are a number of issues that practitioners have to consider, the ways in which we frame events, the ways in which we make decisions. We often do not have enough information to make a scientific decision, we have to make a professional one. This is sometimes based upon best available information, and lessons learned about approaches to care through past experience and group discovery.

Depending upon your expectations of professional education, EBL may seem less satisfying than PBL. It seems to offer less authoritative outcomes, even if the lessons learned within the process extend to group skills and ways of investigating. You may consider it more authentic to nursing and nurse education, precisely because it attends to aesthetic matters and how we might approach care. In part, such reactions are to do with the varied nature of health care practice, and in part they concern themselves with your style of learning and the way in which you understand the world. You may not believe that the world can be understood always in terms of facts, or conversely that to deal always with impressions is really rather unprofessional. Either way, engaging in EBL study will help you clarify your views as well as potentially discover information that you can use to reconsider practice. At the close of this chapter I make the case to you, while not all of health care is amenable to research evidence, most of it may be open to either problem- or enquiry-based learning. It is arguable that what is learned through enquiry-based learning may be superior to personal reflection precisely because it has been challenged by colleagues and debated within a study group.

4 Using a Scaffold for Inquiries

To close Part I of this book it is now appropriate to look at the use of a 'scaffold' to facilitate your inquiries, both those associated with problem- and enquiry-based learning. One the commonest anxieties associated with PBL/EBL study centre upon understanding the nature of the problem (PBL) or the focus for inquiries (EBL). Within the early modules of PBL programmes of study, the problem may be dictated by tutor notes or instructions. The group facilitator explicitly states the issues that are likely to be important. In subsequent modules, and as you become more adept at PBL investigations, trigger information may become rather more meagre. Your study group is expected to shape your own inquiry, determining the nature of the problem and first inquiries for yourselves. Within EBL scoping the inquiry necessarily involves considering what sorts of information might be relevant, as well as where this could be obtained.

There is therefore a case, at least in circumstances where you find it difficult to get into an investigation, for considering the use of a scaffold to help prompt questions and to encourage speculation about what could be important. The term scaffold simply refers to ways of thinking about a problem or an investigation, which help you to consider its different dimensions. Scaffolds are simply a prop (Spouse, 1998). That is, they have no intrinsic purpose in and of themselves, but provide tools with which to start your own investigative work. A successful scaffold encourages you to think laterally about the problem. Importantly, it should not unduly constrain your thinking about the investigation. Rather, as the artist may need encouragement to make the first brush stroke upon a blank canvas, so the problem-solver or inquirer may need a modest assistance with imagining where to make a start.

Historically, nurses have employed models of nursing as scaffolds to help them think about care (Griffiths, 1998; Tierney, 1998). Unfortunately, many such models have constrained nursing thought, dictating how nursing *should* be construed. There has been a tendency for practitioners to own allegiance to one or other theorist and to argue the importance of a particular perspective upon nursing. In this chapter therefore the scaffold that is proposed will not be based upon a model of nursing. Rather, it will highlight several elements of nursing which might start to suggest useful lines of inquiry, and which may facilitate critical thinking in your study group. Chenoweth (1998) and Brookfield (1987) both emphasize the importance of critical thinking within life, and both acknowledge the value of exercises or activities that prompt this at the start of study.

Our rather simple scaffold has been developed from a distance learning programme module on exploring nursing practice through PBL means (Price, 1998a) and through subsequent practice investigations conducted with midwives (Price and Price, 2000). It admits different philosophies and approaches to practice, while enabling practitioners to think about areas within which a problem may exist or issues that could help them clarify nursing approaches further (EBL). It consists of asking questions about the nature of knowledge used within practice, the frames of reference that guide how we approach practice situations, decision-making steps that are often used in clinical settings and the ways in which research evidence or theory have influenced practice to date.

In Figure 4.1, reference is made to the inquisitive approach necessary within each of the scaffold areas. We will now work our way through each of these in turn, offering illustrations of what each might have to offer. Because your own investigations may occur with a wide variety of different fields of practice, the illustrations will be eclectic, offering examples that I hope will be of interest to a range of readers. In describing the scaffold it is important to remember that this is not meant to dictate all aspects of your investigation. On the contrary, once inquiries have been prompted, it is often more important to leave the scaffold behind, following the leads that seem most fruitful to the study group.

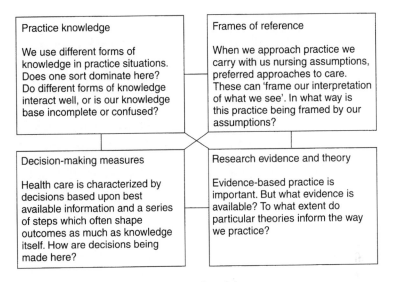

Figure 4.1   A scaffold for PBL/EBL inquiries

Source: After Price (1998a); Price and Price (2000)

PRACTICE KNOWLEDGE

Consider the following quotes from nurses working within several different settings. These imply a number of things about the nature of practice knowledge, many of which could be significant in a problem analysis or practice inquiry:

> People are sometimes funny but when you meet patients and their wives for the first time, you do have to form impressions about how they are. You sense whether they are fretful, angry, intelligent or passive. I think this information is the stuff of nursing work – it's what you have to work with if you're going to make a success of what you tell patients and what you do for them.
>
> (Raymet, talking about hospital admission interviews)

> I feel happiest when I can tell relatives something concrete about the surgery and the rehabilitation that follows. I'm the sort of person who keeps a notebook in my pocket, so I'm always whipping that out and doing sketches to show them what is involved in stoma surgery.
>
> (Jane, stoma care specialist)

> Some nurses are especially valuable because they have this knack of knowing how to get things done, how to get the best out of the system for their patients. OK, they know how to make referrals, but they're brilliant too at knowing how to approach others, so that there will be a helpful response.
>
> (Donald, care of older adults)

Eraut (1990) has pointed out that practitioners often make use of tacit knowledge. That is, they employ a wealth of knowledge which is rarely discussed, but which is drawn upon repeatedly because it has been found to be useful. Tacit knowledge is knowledge which has passed the utility test – it works in practice, enabling nurses and others to make sense of the situations they encounter. Where such knowledge becomes strongly embedded, so that it habitually influences the way in which nurses understand patients, problems and needs, then it can be called a personal construct (Buckenham, 1998). Personal constructs are extremely powerful, short-hand ways of understanding the world. They are powerful precisely because it would otherwise prove exhausting to interpret each and every new situation on an individual basis (see Price, 1987). Health care practitioners employ short-hand accounts of what is happening in order to manage the information overload that comes their way each day.

The above quotations refer to what Eraut (1990) has described as people, empirical and process knowledge, respectively. You develop a store of knowledge about people, how they feel, how they are likely to react, what they may worry about or need, based partly upon what you would think or feel in that situation yourself, and partly upon experiences built up over time. People knowledge is in large part aesthetic and fuels much of what we mean when they talk about practice intuition. It is used to guess how best to approach strangers in different professional settings and how to deal with issues when there is no obvious *correct* answer. Empirical knowledge refers to what the practitioner thinks of as 'facts'. It is often based upon a science where information is considered indisputable or at least highly respectable. Empirical knowledge is often thought of as superior knowledge with which to work. In this example, Jane is relying upon knowledge of anatomy and physiology, of surgical procedures to increase her confidence in helping patients. The process knowledge that Donald admires seems to be of two kinds. There are the formal processes that have to be understood and used (referrals within hospital, for instance) and the informal processes – interpersonal ways of winning arguments, persuading others and getting a better deal for a client.

Just why it is worth thinking about practice knowledge as part of PBL or EBL is because we often need to understand the knowledge in use to appreciate the situation. The knowledge that an investigator might imagine is being used may not be the same as the knowledge that is being used. Knowledge employed, and how it is applied within practice, may be hidden from the casual observer. By considering practice knowledge within relevant contexts it may be possible to ascertain whether you are using the most valid knowledge, whether you are employing particular forms of knowledge more and whether you are aware of how you typically think about situations. This is nicely illustrated within an example from child health nursing where the investigator made notes about the habitual use of knowledge concerning child abuse and parenting (see Box 4.1).

Box 4.1   Investigation notes: child-abusing parents

Faced with the need to sum up parents quickly within the care unit, nurses rely upon the ways in which parents dress, the way in which they interact with children and the way they talk about parenting experiences to identify parents who need careful monitoring. They cannot ask the parent how they view discipline or chastisement or whether they love their child, because they would simply receive a conventional response. Instead, they become concerned about the slovenly dressed (less capable) and the immaculately dressed (too busy to care) and wonder whether this parent values the relationship with his or her child. In particular, they examine the way parents cope with unexpected child behaviour, their own or that of others on the unit. Do these parents contain their anger or surprise, or is there a sudden and brisk response? The smack withheld may say as much as the smack administered. Parents, who dismiss their child, describing typical traits and habits, observing that 'kids are like that', may also come under suspicion. Anything that suggests a lack of respect for the individuality of the child is scrutinized.

In this investigation the nurse discovers that the nurses have a working profile of the child-abusing parent type and that this helps to determine whether parents are considered 'colleague carers' or visitors that need to be monitored. It comes from an EBL investigation of how nurses interact with lay carers, deciding what to expect of them. Whether the practice knowledge is well founded or adequate may be a matter for debate, but here it does identify what information is being used to formulate approaches to lay carers. Understanding the tacit knowledge of practitioners assists the study group to start describing the general approach of nurses (in certain situations) to professional/lay care interaction.

Practice knowledge offers a scaffold to investigations therefore because we can start to ask important questions about how nurses think and approach situations. The following list is not exhaustive, but may serve to encourage debate and new lines of inquiry:

- Do we understand the knowledge being used here?
- Do the practitioners think about their knowledge use (assumptions)?
- Do all parties understand knowledge in the same way?
- Does knowledge change from situation to situation, if so, how and at what points?
- Do different elements of knowledge conflict, leaving the nurse in a quandary about what to think?
- Are there problems with this knowledge (is it ethical or professional)?
- Where does the knowledge come from – is there a prime source?

Sometimes the availability, use or abuse of knowledge are at the heart of a practice problem. Individual practitioners may use access to certain forms of knowledge to secure or retain power. In other instances there is a shortfall of the most modern and well-informed forms of knowledge, for instance, where practice is based upon custom rather than quizzical reflection or research.

FRAMES OF REFERENCE

Some years ago the British police produced a poster advertisement, which featured a young Afro-Caribbean man dressed in shirt and jeans running in front of a young white Caucasian male, dressed in a police uniform. The poster challenged the viewer to interpret what was happening in this scene and then, in small print below, explained that both men were, in fact, police officers, in hot pursuit of another male (out of picture). This cleverly designed poster highlights a number of things about what we can call the frames of reference that people use to interpret situations. The first is that a frame of reference may be erroneous and influenced by prejudice or bias. The young Afro-Caribbean man was not the criminal, but a fellow police officer. An individual examining the poster might be tempted to assume that the uniformed officer was chasing this individual, based upon racial prejudices, or at the very least, an ignorance that Afro-Caribbean men contribute their services as plain clothes officers within the police service. The second lesson to be learned is that social situations (including those relating to health) are often constructed. That is, individuals ascribe meanings to what they see, and irrespective of whether their perceptions are sound, use these to direct their behaviour and their future responses to similar situations.

The significance of this short detour from health care is that frames of reference, those held by individuals, groups or organizations, may form part of a problem, practice or could contribute to a solution. Michel Foucault, an influential philosopher, has highlighted the importance of such ascribed meanings and their power to frame a reality, enticing or forcing others to see situations in a similar way (Foucault, 1990). This is nicely illustrated in a study by Parker *et al.* (1992) who researched the nursing shift handover within hospitals. Parker and Wiltshire observed how the account of patients, their progress, needs and behaviour during the last shift influenced nurses coming on to shift next. Patients who were considered unco-operative, demanding or needful would continue to be seen in this light for the next shift, at least, unless a radical change in their condition intervened. Patients might become labelled over successive shifts and particular care approaches reinforced.

Frames of reference shape the ways in which health care is delivered and may or may not be understood by those individuals delivering the care. In some instances the frame of reference is expressed corporately (for instance, as a philosophy of care), in others it is expressed tacitly (as in the way the situation was described by nurses going off shift, to those coming on shift, in Parker *et al.*'s work). Because frames of reference express what

---

Box 4.2   Observations from the casualty department

It is Friday evening and following a RTA (Road Traffic Accident) a pedestrian has died in casualty. The staff nurse who supported the resuscitation effort is distraught and needs a short break before resuming the rest of her night shift. Sister X makes time to comfort and support the nurse, using the staff room to help her rehearse her feelings about events and efforts to save the unfortunate victim of a drunk driving incident. Afterwards, Sister X explains at length how she deals with sudden death, and managing shock and personal evaluation of practice in Christian ways. She is a deeply committed Christian herself and finds it useful to evaluate care efforts in such terms. In this instance the staff nurse has no particular religious faith. The staff nurse reports some hours later that she found the support from Sister X uncomfortable but regrets not having explained this to her.

---

practitioners take as a given, as custom and practice, they often deserve investigation as part of a PBL or EBL study. Frames of reference frequently express nursing ideologies (see Chapter 1), but they may also express other convictions too (see Box 4.2).

In this example from an investigation on what constitutes good practice in the support of professional colleagues, the study group begins a new line of inquiry concerning ethnic or religious norms and expressions of help. The investigator was alerted to the significance of her observations in practice because the group had already talked about the ways in which individuals have the power to define situations. At the outset it was argued that this was sometimes good (others not being ready or willing to take this responsibility) and sometimes problematic (because definitions could prove intrusive for others). By exploring frames of reference as one possible aspect of colleague support, investigators were assisted to focus their observations in fresh new ways. Instead of asking whether this incident proved an adequate support for the nurse, in terms of space, time, physical comfort, the investigator questioned whether there was always a fit between what practitioners needed and what was provided. The way in which this sister frames 'support of colleagues' appeared to have limited what she was able to achieve. Significantly, the question then arose, was the sister aware of this limitation and were there sensitive ways of helping her to discover alternative support approaches?

Frames of reference can represent a problem within practice, or explain why care is expressed in particular ways. This is as true with regard to large-scale initiatives as it is to day-to-day practice. For instance, consider the approach taken towards nursing leadership within a particular health care Trust. Within this Trust, leadership is conceived of as distinct from management, and designed to promote self-confidence and professional growth among all staff, not simply senior officers. As a result, the hospital staff development team use a particular frame of reference when they select staff for leadership development programmes and measure the practitioners' success in specific ways. Selection, education and progress assessment are fundamentally framed by what the team believes leadership to consist of. Were such an approach to come into conflict with other stakeholders, perhaps senior managers, or other training agencies, then the frame of reference represents an important part of the problem analysis. It is not that one particular frame of reference is right or wrong. Rather, within such situations it may be that frames of reference are in conflict and that stakeholders need to understand their assumptions and those of others, before a resolution can be sought.

DECISION-MAKING MEASURES

Decision-making is at the heart of many practice investigations and problem analyses. It is especially important because the outcomes may be highly significant (leading to life or death) and because in the main, practitioners have imperfect information upon which to make their decisions (Cioffi, 1998). Decision-making is extremely stressful for nurses, sometimes conducted in teams and sometimes as an individual practitioner. The time frame of decisions varies widely, from those associated with incremental support measures for chronically ill patients (made over years) to those completed within minutes (for instance, in

association with a threatened suicide). While practitioners typically make the best decision possible under given circumstances,
they may be held accountable for the outcomes long afterwards.
For example, the decision that a midwife makes while supporting
a woman in childbirth may be critically revisited many years later
through a court of law, if the child was later proven to be brain
damaged. Were the decisions made then the right decisions, as
indicated by hospital policy or protocol, and with regard to what
a reasonable practitioner, up to date with research evidence and
a concern for the client would do? Cases of negligence rest upon
professional knowledge and the ways in which practitioners use
this knowledge to choose courses of action (Green, 1999).

The ways in which decisions are made, and actions elected, are
a legitimate focus of interest within problem- and enquiry-based
learning. This is not necessarily because care has gone wrong in
some way (and blame is being apportioned). It may be important
because care is working extremely well, and the study group
need to understand just why care is so successful. It is easy to be
complacent about success and to lose the opportunity to enhance
achievement, simply because no problems have arisen.

A number of texts have been written on clinical decision-
making (e.g. Winfield, 1998; Young, 2002). One useful source
comes from Dowie and Elstein's edited volume, *Professional
Judgement: A Reader in Clinical Decision Making* (Dowie and Elstein,
1988). In this volume different approaches to decision-making
are reviewed, including those which employ computer modelling.
Contrasts are drawn between inductive processes (i.e. asking
questions such as, 'What is happening here?' in order to identify
a sensitive response) and deductive processes (where hypotheses
are formed about what is likely to happen if we elect certain
courses of action). Elstein and Bordage (1988) usefully describe
how clinical decision-making comprises a number of components
(see Figure 4.2).

Decisions are based upon available information, and may
therefore be tentative at first and refined later. The practitioner
collects cues, that is, bits of information that seem to suggest
what *might* be happening, and what *may* be of concern. Whether
the practitioner notices or gathers the right cues or enough cues
will help to determine whether the clinical decision is well
founded. Having gathered as many cues together as possible, the
practitioner then needs to interpret what these add up to, what

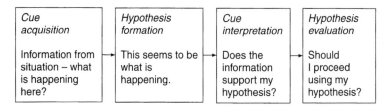

Figure 4.2   Decision-making components

Source: Adapted from Elstein and Bordage (1988)

they represent. Lazarus and Folkman (1984) have described just this sort of appraisal process with regard to people under stress. They try to assess whether a phenomenon represents a threat, and if so, whether they feel able to cope with this. Clinicians interpret cues in order to ascertain the clinical significance of what is happening and to suggest whether something urgent needs to be done.

While it seems unlikely that nurses and others routinely formulate formal hypotheses of the scientific type, they do regularly decide what a situation means and what this signifies regarding an appropriate action. The plan of action is possibly tentative and subject to early adjustment in the light of new information. This said, it is still a working hypothesis of what is required now and what might help in this situation. It usually involves imagining what the benefits or the shortfalls of action or inaction are likely to be. It sometimes involves debating the merits of different courses of action and whether the selection of one precludes other opportunities later on. Finally, with access to further observations, tests or investigations, or the response of the patient, the practitioner evaluates whether the cues were adequately understood and whether hypotheses seemed sound.

Cioffi and Markham (1997) conducted a research study into the ways in which midwives made decisions with women during labour. They considered the ways in which different cues were weighed, in order to ascertain the level of risk that a woman faced. This was an important consideration given that there were pressures not to intervene prematurely (women sought a natural childbirth) and pressures to contain risks (either to mother or baby). Intervention might reduce or even negate risk if action was timely and effective. In studies such as this, the importance of decision-making in avoiding or creating problems becomes apparent. The ways in which midwives weighed the significance of different cues (with greater emphasis upon physiological signs) helped to define how they saw risk during labour.

Within a problem- or enquiry-based learning project it may be fruitful to begin investigation with the ways in which decisions are made in practice. Decision-making may prove to be the central issue in a practice, or the focus of a problem. In the following example from a problem-based learning project on managing risk within the burns unit, students were invited to consider not only what the risk factors were, but how these were measured (Box 4.3). Initially the group began their study by learning more about hypovolaemic shock, the nature of infection and the challenge associated with pain management. They quickly appreciated, however, that it was the management of combined risks, the ways in which clinicians make decisions that were most important in how theory was turned into action.

Box 4.3   Student reflection (risk in the burns unit)

I don't think that our tutor expected us to focus so intensely upon decision-making when we started this investigation. We'd worked our way through understanding the physiological problems and got the hang of those cleanly enough. Then, though, Cheryl said, 'So you want to manage pain, but you need to consider what opiates do to the base line obs, the patients' respiration. How does the burns team get those decisions right?' Well, that was it, we were on the trail and interrogated the doctors and senior nurses in order to try and understand the decisions they took. I suppose we all wanted to feel secure before we faced such decisions. We got to the bottom of it using case examples – decisions that had already been made. I only wish that decision-making had been on the agenda earlier. I think we could have got further with this one.

Decision-making, together with frames of reference and practice knowledge suggest places to look within an investigation and prompt a range of questions that could be posed early within the study. Here is a sample of the questions, suggested through the scaffold that might be asked about decision-making:

- What cues seem important in this decision-making process?
- How are cues interpreted and by whom?
- To what extent does the decision-making process involve consultation?
- Who is responsible for the various aspects of decision-making work? Is it the same person, if not, how do they communicate?
- How are hypotheses formed? On what do they focus?
- How does the clinician know care is appropriate?
- What alerts the practitioner to make a new decision (perhaps to reverse a previous one)?
- How does intuition contribute to decision-making?

Asking questions such as these, not only do you begin to indicate what the focus of your inquiry will be, but you begin to suggest what sort of data might be important and where this could be found. For example, asking questions about consultation in decision-making could conceivably be emotive. Practitioners are anxious about how others might judge their decision-making style. There may be information offered by practitioners (claimed consultation) and that provided by observation (either supporting or refuting what the practitioners say). In a study it may be necessary to gather both sorts of information in order to decide whether decision-making is at the heart of a problem associated with judging cardiac rehabilitation – how far and how fast?

RESEARCH EVIDENCE OR PROFESSIONAL THEORY?

There has been a long-running debate about the interface between theory or research evidence and practice (Retsas, 2000). Some common concerns attend here, most notably that practitioners do not make critical and effective use of theory or research evidence in practice. The theory–practice gap (what you should do or would do, in theory, and what happens in clinical practice) has been one of the primary drivers for the introduction of PBL and EBL approaches within nurse education. Practitioners are often criticized for not using available research evidence, based upon the relatively naïve assumption that research evidence is easy to interpret and apply within different contexts. In practice, research evidence is of different types and involves different evaluative criteria (see Table 4.1).

Table 4.1   Types of research evidence

Research paradigm	Type of evidence	Evaluative criteria
Positivist (descriptive surveys, experimental/ quasi-experimental designs, randomized clinical control trials)	Usually quantitative, but with emphasis upon testing a theory or hypothesis, examining the impact of interventions upon outcomes or measuring a situation or condition	Validity/reliability control of the research environment and research variables, questions about the size and representativeness of the sample
Naturalistic (interpretive or constructive in emphasis). (Several forms of Ethnography/ Phenomenology Grounded Theory/ Case Study research and Ethnomethodology)	Usually qualitative data, with an emphasis upon illuminating reality explaining phenomena within a particular context. The world is seen as complex, especially with regard to the meanings used by individuals to appreciate their situation and select appropriate behaviour	Authenticity – does this account seem an authentic representation of what respondents offered (judged by checking the audit trail, the account of how researchers gathered and analysed data)? Does this account seem familiar/realistic given my own local practice/ experience?
Critical theory (Marxist or feminist-inspired, addressing the political/ideological nature of knowledge or practice). Action research is frequently used as the design	May be qualitative or quantitative but typically includes reference to the need to appreciate the situation of the disadvantaged, to right or wrong or promote change	Authenticity and audit trail are used here (see above). Validity is, however, also evaluated against the philosophical/ ideological values made explicit (as a given) within the study

Source: After Price (2000a)

Table 4.1 illustrates just how sophisticated research evaluation has to be. Whereas once upon a time nurses were taught that all research was evaluated in terms of validity and reliability, they are now advised that these notions themselves betray a series of assumptions about the health care world. Paradigms (world-views about the nature of the world and what should be taken as true about what is experienced) vary. It has been pointed out that we now practise within what has been called the 'postmodernist' world (e.g. Robinson, 2000). Within this world there are competing accounts of reality.

Positivism, for instance, emphasizes empirical truths, the importance of being able to predict or even control outcomes, because the researcher or practitioner deals with what were deemed to be facts. Naturalism, in contrast, emphasizes the world of meanings, the ways in which human beings construct an account of reality that is just as pervasive and powerful as empirical facts. It is argued that nurses work with the meanings that patients and others ascribe to health and disease – defining what they mean by 'illness' (Thorsteinsson, 2002). Critical theorists in turn argue that knowledge can never be philosophically neutral. The very way in which we select, gather and use knowledge, in research, in practice, is inherently political. There is often no objective truth, only a defensible position, and researchers should therefore nail their colours to a mast against which their findings can then be evaluated.

This poses a number of important questions regarding the place of research evidence within practice. Some of these have been part of the traditional discussion about why research evidence is not applied but others are rather more searching:

• What research evidence is available within this area and where is it sourced (the source needs to be accessible and trustworthy). Some nurses might also argue that it needs to be professionally 'home grown' rather than borrowed from other professions.
• Does the research evidence fit with the practice context (research evidence might not translate well across ethnic/geographical/health care system boundaries)?
• Is it easy to understand the type of research evidence on offer?
• Does this type of research evidence correspond with the assumptions and values of the practitioners within the investigative study area?

- Is this type of research evidence considered valuable within the wider multidisciplinary setting (for example, doctors have historically been educated to value positivist research evidence above all others)? They are much more circumspect about the value of naturalistic or critical theory-inspired 'qualitative' research.
- Does the research evidence offer clear conclusions, either recommendations for practice or useful illumination of what it is important for practitioners to consider as they plan change?

It is relatively easy to ascribe problems in the uptake of research to the complexities of research evidence, the prejudice or ignorance of practitioners or the lack of support for change at higher levels within the organization. Within a problem- or enquiry-based learning investigation, however, it may be necessary to ask rather more profound questions. Box 4.4 is an extract from a discussion between two EBL investigators who are interested in what constitutes quality enhancement within cancer care. They have both agreed that research evidence might contribute to an improved quality of treatment and care for patients, but that medical and nursing staff are by no means agreed on what evidence should be employed in practice development, or how it could be used.

Box 4.4   Asking questions about research evidence

Carmel: Looking at the research available on chemotherapy side effects and their management, I think you can place it into one of two piles. You have the material that's all about managing symptoms, controlling the problem. You know, the stuff about reducing nausea and limiting hair loss. Then you have the other research which is all about fatigue and hope, sustaining a quality of life that patients think is worth having. The second sort of research doesn't seem to assume what is best for the patient.

Ben: I don't think those researchers assume that we can solve the patients' problems. All we can do with some aspects of the cancer experience is understand it a bit more sensitively and help the patients to find answers that work for them.

> *Carmel*: I don't think the two sorts of research are mutually exclusive. I mean, they both have a place and patients could get better care if we used both. The problem though is that that some staff will only value the problem-solving research, and dismiss the other material as 'nice to know'. The qualitative material doesn't seem to offer a clear steer on what we should do.
>
> *Ben*: There's some prejudice there I agree, but we're still left with the challenge – how do you use the qualitative data research so that it chimes with the problem-solving stuff? How do you get our friends to value that sort of adjustment in front of the patient? If they don't respect the other initiatives, the patient won't feel confident using our help.
>
> *Carmel*: We need some sort of best practice approaches, based upon recognition of the qualitative research. We have to decide whether it fits here and to what extent it informs how we approach care.
>
> *Ben*: And we also have to explain our thinking to the doubters.

What Carmel and Ben discuss in this extract might be regarded as research cultures. Two cultures operate within their practice area, one strongly positivist in nature and the other naturalist. The EBL project itself seems to be steered by critical theory concerns, to make the lot of the patient much better, through a more integrated approach to support. Within PBL/EBL inquiries it is often necessary to examine such cultures, and to resist the temptation to simply blame others for a poor research evidence uptake. Research cultures need to be understood, and if change is to be promoted, then consideration needs to be given to how this can be strategically conceived. In this example, to simply confront colleagues with the error of their thinking seems unlikely to work. A better solution might be to encourage colleagues to applaud 'best practice approaches' where they acknowledge there is as yet no definitive, problem-solving solution. By analysing the research evidence–practice interface at a deeper level, investigators have a greater chance of recommending action that promotes change in the future.

THEORY AND PRACTICE

So far we have discussed the research evidence–practice interface. Theory and practice also benefit from a similar critical evaluation. Nurses use a variety of theories, or bits of theory to reinforce their practice decisions and to help them feel they are practising professionally (Fealy, 1999). Many of these theories are themselves devised within a paradigm, a world-view about health, illness and health care practice. Consider the following observations from nurses who are talking about their own use of theory within practice:

> I've always found Peplau's theory useful within my work. When you stop and think about it, we are strangers to patients and no matter how clever or skilful you are, the relationship you begin with that patient is the medium through which you show what you can do. Get the relationship wrong and nothing much else can work.
>
> (Phil, community mental health worker)

> I remember reading about the theory, which suggests that our bodies produce a natural supply of endorphins, chemicals that help us feel good and manage discomfort. When someone is dying, that natural supply is used up, so we use analgesics to supplement what they would otherwise have. It helps me resist the arguments of others who say that opiates will damage the patient's quality of life by making them sleepy all the time.
>
> (Imogen, oncology care nurse)

> Some theories really irritate me. I work with renal dialysis patients and the stuff that Maslow wrote about a hierarchy of needs just doesn't work with chronically ill folk. They meet self-esteem needs like eating or drinking things their friends do, even though they know this makes them ill. Patients aren't rational and they don't always deal with physiological or safety needs first.
>
> (Wesley, renal dialysis unit)

In Phil's case he talks in approving terms of a nursing care model that was devised several decades ago (Peplau, 1994). Peplau's work has been influential with many practitioners but what is important for our discussion here is that there is a good fit between Phil's philosophy of care and that espoused in Peplau's theory. This can be summed as professional relationships being therapeutic in and of themselves. The inter-professional relationship is not simply the medium for other work to be done (e.g. history taking), it is itself capable of helping patients feel better. Within an inquiry it is worth examining whether particular theories are widely used and whether the philosophy of the practitioners and the philosophy implicit within the theory are in close agreement. In situations where multiple theories are in use, or where there is a poor philosophical match between theory and practice, there may be problems in making care coherent. Where, however, the theory in use by practitioners seems out of kilter with health care developments, the expressed needs of the consumer, even a widely subscribed to theory may be problematic. Consider, for instance, theories that portray the patient as an equal partner and decision-maker within rehabilitation. Where large numbers of patients prefer to see themselves as more passive recipients of health care teaching, this theory could become problematic.

Imogen presents another aspect of the theory–practice interface. In this case she is reporting a borrowed theory (from physiology) and one that she can but vaguely describe. Many practitioners subscribe to bits of theory, some of which may be applied out of context. In this case Imogen uses the theory as a support for her own philosophical approach to analgesia within palliative care. Theory is used to justify an approach, which in this instance seems to imply that analgesia supplements the body, and that if this is titrated correctly it need not damage the patient's quality of life. What is important here is that theories are not always adopted, lock, stock and barrel within practice. Individuals and groups may select bits of theory to suit a local purpose or preferred care approach. Such an eclectic selection of concepts can often work well for patients and practitioners, but in some other instances, incomplete, misconstrued or misapplied theory can be at the centre of a problem.

Wesley's experience of Maslow's theory, a hierarchy of needs (Maslow, 1987) is instructive for other reasons. In this example Wesley demonstrates a quizzical attitude towards theory. His practice experience constantly challenges the theory he has remembered from college. Maslow wrote about motivation, suggesting that needs of different order drove motivation, suggesting to individuals how they should behave. Wesley correctly observes that sometimes patients try to meet higher order needs (self-esteem), before they have secured lower order needs (safety). What is important here is that theory is critically examined, before it is applied. Like research, it is tested for its utility – whether it fits within practice. It is important to examine situations to see whether theory is understood well and whether practitioners have a discriminating attitude towards the use of theory. At one extreme, a slavish adoption of theory can be detrimental to patients and practitioners alike. Practice situations are made to fit the theory, and care delivered to a formula. At the other extreme, the practitioner is left without norms or principles. Because theory (or research evidence) is unavailable or unclear, he or she acts in situation to situation, managing stress as well as possible.

We can now sum up some useful scaffold questions that might be asked about the relationship between theory and practice within an investigation. As before, these are illustrative and certainly not prescribed. However, one or more of these might provide useful leads for your future inquiry:

- Does theory have an influence here? If so, which theories are important and how are they being used?
- Is theory absent here? Does this matter?
- Is there a coherent theory in use here, or multiple bits of theory? Does this matter?
- How is theory being employed by practitioners – to reinforce their practice, or to challenge their thinking?
- Where has theory come from? Is this up to date and relevant now?
- Do the theories in use by practitioners coincide with the theories in use by clients? Is this problematic?
- Do practitioners have a clear idea of how theory could be used in this context, or is there literally a gap in interpretation/ application?

CONCLUSION

Scaffolds require cautious use within health care, a field where frameworks have all too readily become mantras. Nevertheless, within PBL/EBL projects, where areas for investigation may at first seem unclear, it does seem useful to have a scaffold available.

Practice problems are often a mix of issues associated with knowledge, frames of reference, the ways in which decisions are made and the extent to which research evidence or theory are employed. Health care practice often involves selecting particular combinations of knowledge and theory in order to reach an important end. While every investigation will involve a unique blend of knowledge, theory (perhaps research evidence), decision-making and frames of reference, it seems likely that we will need to work with most of these concepts.

One of the greatest benefits of problem- and enquiry-based learning is that it makes us conscious of how we understand practice and why we behave as we do. PBL/EBL approaches force us to be more conscious of that which might otherwise be taken for granted. Reflexive practitioners are typified by their metacognition. That is, they are more aware of what they are doing, their motives and why they employ particular resources or approaches. Using a scaffold within your own inquiries will, I argue, acquaint you with practice issues at a deeper level. You will think more intensively, reflectively and within a great deal more introspection. Scaffold questions might offer suggestions where to start, but beyond that they will also help you to think about the conduct of your inquiry. Asking questions such as these, it will be difficult to avoid thinking about what you believe or feel, what you value or aspire to. In short, as a PBL or EBL investigator you will become a more thoughtful and strategic practitioner.

Part II

MAKING INQUIRIES

5 ACCESSING AND GATHERING INFORMATION

Accessing and gathering information represent a significant part of the effort associated with problem- and enquiry-based learning. It is not, however, simply a 'go for' activity. It is important to plan the information gathering process and to consider just where and how the most useful information might be obtained. Time is always at a premium, and your group facilitator will be keen to ensure that you learn something through the process of information access and retrieval. As has been argued in Part I, PBL and EBL are not solely concerned with finding answers to questions, it is about discovering new ways to learn and collaborate. In the end, the group process skills that you will develop are those that are likely to serve you in the longer term. The answers to problems are often transient, practice moves on. The skills of inquiry and analysis though are potentially lifelong learning benefits.

Having reviewed the problem case study, or scoped the subject that your study group will investigate information gathering follows next. Your group facilitator should have helped you clarify just what you wish to find out, and the scaffold described in Chapter 4 may well assist you. You have either volunteered or agreed to make 'certain inquiries', either on your own or in association with another group member. As you contemplate this work a number of considerations need to be taken into account (see Figure 5.1).

If you are to be a strategic inquirer you need to work with the time available to you for this stage of the investigation. Group facilitators or study group chairs normally set a date by which time information is once again pooled. If you are completing this project part-time, you will need to consider what time you can allocate to the investigation. You will certainly need to anticipate just how long it might take to gather information from different

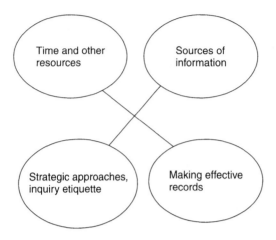

Figure 5.1 Planning information gathering

sources. For example, obtaining more obscure references through a library can take several weeks if this involves an inter-library loan. It may be more appropriate to work with other resources that are more accessible. It is well worth setting down what you think your time resources and personal capacities are, indicating what sources of information you hope to use, and then consulting the group facilitator to check whether he or she thinks you have set yourself a manageable task. This is not cheating. Project management skills are often brought to PBL and EBL by facilitators, and they are certainly skills that can be learned rather more quickly (and less painfully) by asking for advice (Hilterbrand, 1997).

The various possible sources of information form the bulk of this chapter and the one that follows. Different sources of advice, however, have different strengths and limitations (see Table 5.1). You will need to decide which sources fit best with the type of information that you seek, and which will be most accessible or manageable within the available time frame. In one investigation you may access several sources of information, however, beware – a project that is well scoped, and carefully managed, should not require you to access multiple sources within tight time frames. Where a problem or situation needs to be understood from several different angles it is often more appropriate to leave investigators to explore one source of information, albeit intensively. Thereafter

Table 5.1 Information sources, strengths and limitations

Source	Strengths	Limitations
Documents	Often authoritative. Accessible if local. Policies/protocols may be open to repeated scrutiny or loan	Slow to access, if from an external source. May involve literature searching (? subject well defined). May involve technical or statistical data, requiring further analysis
People	May provide expert and local knowledge. May be enthusiastic and suggest additional sources. May assist with interim interpretation of the problem/situation	People are stakeholders in situations and may provide an eclectic perspective. Senior staff have limited time and access, maybe through a secretary or receptionist. Excess intrusion might prejudice them against helping you or colleagues in the future
Practice observation	Locally, very accessible. Heightens your awareness of practice issues	Need to observe ethical principles and to make clear records
Field trips	Observation in centres of excellence, opportunity to compare and contrast practices (fresh perspective)	Time-consuming/costly to arrange. Information may not transfer well between contexts

the group can pool the investigations of different group members upon the subject.

Different skills are needed (and developed) through gathering information from different sources. For example, gathering documentary information involves library skills and the ability to code information from text that was not written to your specific purpose. Information gathering from people involves interviewing skills, while observation in practice requires skills of negotiation and record-making. If you are working in an investigative pair, check whether your partner has any of these particular skills and work to this advantage. Don't be afraid to ask your colleague for advice, or in turn, if you are the more experienced partner, to explain your thinking. Take a look at this reflection from one investigator:

> I suddenly realized that Jane hadn't ever worked at getting past a receptionist to speak to a GP before. I'd done it many times as a sales rep. I took the lead for that reason, but I had Jane listen in to the way I made my telephone calls. GPs are busy people and receptionists are protective. I wanted everyone to feel OK about any help given at the end, so I worded my requests very carefully indeed.
>
> (Pauline, nurse practitioner)

GATHERING INFORMATION FROM PEOPLE

Problem- and enquiry-based learning has the potential to exhaust and frustrate clinical experts, at least where investigators handle their approach poorly and where they then seem badly organized at interview. The very fact that you target an individual for inquiry usually means that he or she is either considered an expert on a subject, or because he or she has particularly authentic information. Either way, this is likely to mean that the person is in great demand and time will be a precious commodity. For you to succeed with this source of information it will be important to consider all of the following:

- Time constraints (when and for long can these people talk with you?).
- Appreciation of your 'mission' (if the expert does not understand your investigation or its PBL/EBL base, you may need to provide a short briefing).
- Your respondent's feelings or perspective (respondents have their own perspectives, so you will need to inquire sensitively).
- Whether there is an appropriate 'access etiquette'. (It may be necessary to ask permission to conduct interviews. You may be required to contact the nursing/medical director to outline the purpose of your request.)
- What you really want to discover from your interview (often this means a compromise, time will permit only so much information to be gathered).
- What represents an acceptable form of record-making and whether the respondent will see your notes/write up as part of

the access agreement (some respondents are circumspect about audio tape recordings).

Making appointments to see such individuals, it is necessary to agree a clear purpose for your interview and to secure a date, time and location that you can realistically commit to. Respondents quickly become tired of requests to reschedule an interview, although conversely, some of them require patience of you if they are unavoidably delayed themselves. For these reasons it is wise to agree an appointment by telephone or email and to then confirm this in writing, giving details of what you understand has been agreed. Appointments are much more likely to be granted if you promise to stick to an agreed length of interview (say, 30–60 minutes). Thereafter, plan your questions in advance. If the interview seems professionally sensitive and there is time, send a copy of your planned interview questions beforehand. This will reassure your respondent about the focus of your inquiries. Prior to the interview, rehearse what concerns or perspectives you imagine that the respondent may have. While what emerges from interviews often surprise investigators, it is useful to anticipate lines of inquiry that a respondent might feel less comfortable with. Here is an example of planning by an investigator who was going to talk to members of a patient self-help group. The project was on professional and lay care interaction associated with rehabilitation after a cerebrovascular accident.

> Before I went to talk to the group I made a list of all the things I assumed, and all the things that could be sensitive for the group. For instance, on my list of assumptions, prejudices, I suppose, was my feeling that support groups weren't invariably helpful. They didn't always help a couple cope – they might not help folk move beyond the group as a supportive prop. I didn't want to convey this attitude to them, but I did need to understand how they saw their contribution. That's why I changed some of my questions before the interview.
>
> (Gregg, student nurse)

In this example Gregg is thinking ahead, and arguably likely to achieve a richer interview, precisely because he has anticipated the respondent's needs as well as his own before conducting the interview.

INTERVIEW APPROACH

A variety of interview styles *could* be used within PBL/EBL but none of these should be combative. You are not conducting a political interview on television, and should always bear in mind the impression of investigators that you will leave behind with this respondent. In most instances the purpose of a PBL/EBL interview is to increase insight into a situation and thereafter to clarify certain issues regarding that. Interviews therefore move from the general to the specific, from superficial pleasantries towards more searching questions. They always end with thanks expressed to the respondent for his or her time and the opportunity to ask any questions, or to raise any concerns about the interview just completed.

In research textbooks the development of an interview is usually explained in terms of probe questions – that is, questions which encourage the respondent to say more or to clarify a point. Most investigators find these quite difficult to arrange, especially as many of them arise out of the standard questions that they have written down before the interview. In practice, there is a need to manage the level of intrusion into the respondent's world, but to gather useful information. There is a need to decide when to linger upon a topic, or to move on because it has become difficult for the respondent to answer (Price, 2002b). There is also the need to consider how much you (as the investigator) will share your own thoughts and feelings. In human relationships more detailed information is usually only shared on a reciprocal basis. Trust is built up within conversations as individuals swap secrets.

One possible approach to interviewing therefore is to 'ladder' your questions (Price, 2002a). This approach involves ethically managing the interview in terms of its level of intrusion into the respondent's world. The approach is based upon a number of assumptions. The first of these is that people find it easier to discuss what they have done, what they do, than what they think or believe. For example, questions such as 'What did you do next?' are thought to be easier to answer than 'Why did you do that?' or 'What makes you believe that to be the right way to do things?' Investigations into problems do, however, need to involve questions about knowledge and beliefs, so some questions will seem more searching than others. For this reason, they are arranged

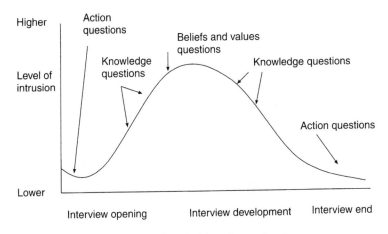

Figure 5.2 Managing intrusion (laddered questions)

later in the interview, and only deployed when the respondent seems more comfortable. This approach can be represented within a simple diagram (see Figure 5.2).

Clearly, Figure 5.2 constitutes a simplified version of interviews, but it does act as a guide to the timing of more intrusive questions. The interview starts with pleasantries, a sharing of action reports (your respondent may indicate what they have 'been up to' while you may describe how your investigation is going). In the early part of the interview you concentrate upon questions that are designed to help the respondents describe the subject, or to outline what he or she does in relation to this. As you do this, monitor facial reactions, body language for any signs of tension (e.g. frowning, tapping of fingers, the adoption of a defensive body posture such as folding of arms). Provided that you both remain comfortable, it is then possible to ask some more searching questions relating to the knowledge that a respondent uses as part of his or her work or understanding of the problem. Here are three examples of these:

So what led you to understand that the patient was changing her mind about this form of treatment?

What is it about TENS therapy that makes it useful for these patients?

What helps you decide when to say something, when to intervene?

What is common to questions like these is that the respondent needs to explain the underlying rationale of action or perspective. The respondent reflects on his or her knowledge and how it is used. This is more intrusive than action questions, so once again it is important to monitor the respondent's reactions to your questions. Provided that you have thought carefully about what you want to share from your own experience or perspective, it can also be fruitful after the respondent has answered to offer a reflection of your own (once again at the knowledge level, see example below): 'I've found that patient's respond to the TENS therapy because they like to feel in control – they can decide what level it runs at. I suppose personal control is important when you're dealing with chronic pain.'

Questions about values, attitudes and beliefs are withheld until the interview is well established and the respondent is answering questions confidently and comfortably. They are only required when you believe that the problem or subject can usefully be understood in philosophical terms. Because questions such as what you believe, why you think this a defensible approach, what you think *should* happen are relatively intimate, it is important to monitor the respondent's reactions to each question. Stand ready to 'ladder down' to easier questions, or move on to other subjects if the line of inquiry seems daunting for the respondent.

Whatever your approach to interviewing, it is important to make clear records. If an audio-tape recording has been agreed, test your equipment before the interview and take along spare batteries, audio-cassettes and a notebook and pencil. Even if I am interviewing using an audio-cassette recorder I keep a notebook, using this to indicate points in the response that I want to return to or new questions or points that might be useful later. Choose an interview location where there is likely to be little or no interruption and ask whether the respondent would feel happy to divert telephone calls for a short period of time. Place the audio-tape recorder equidistant between you, on a firm surface, and at waist height or above. If you are not facing each other for interview, arrange your chair so it is easy to talk towards the microphone. Remember, your questions will be just as important as the answers when you come to interpreting your information.

Students sometimes ask about the relative merits of pre-set questions versus an 'open interview' (Gordon, 1997). While pre-set questions have the merit of reminding you of the areas that you wish to cover, they can also be overtaken by the content of your interview. Respondents sometimes volunteer answers to your later questions in response to your first questions. It is important therefore to remain relatively flexible about interviews, using a list of questions or interview 'areas' to help you steer the interview. For example, reminding yourself that you wish to ask about several different forms of pain relief and that you want to inquire about the 'fit' of these to different pain problems, should help you ensure that your interview retains sufficient breadth. Respondents still have room to offer interesting new information, while your interview continues to have a clear purpose.

GATHERING INFORMATION FROM DOCUMENTS

Within a chapter of this length it is unrealistic to discuss all of the library search skills that should be developed as part of collecting information from documents. For that reason, principles of good library search practice are set out in Box 5.1, before we turn to the examination of documents obtained, either through a library, or through your local health care organization.

Box 5.1 Best practice principles when accessing documents through libraries

- Clarify your search terms, indicate key words that you think might help you to refine your search and discover only the most relevant documents quickly.
- Ask the librarian to show you all the databases on offer. (Libraries often have several and they don't all carry the same information. For example, Psychlit is a database on psychology which might offer some relevant information in nursing.)
- Decide what time span your search will cover. This can help you to limit the size of your search, the volume of information you need to sift through.

Box 5.1   (*continued*)

- Keep careful record of where you searched, including search terms. Avoid the risk of repeating the same search a second time.
- Look at the abstracts of journal articles or books and order only that which seems to have a clear fit (it's expensive and time-consuming to order large volumes of 'may be' photocopies).
- Check with the librarian where a requested item is coming from (if not off the shelf locally). Estimate what time it will take to arrive against your project time frame. Elect whether to proceed with the request.
- When your searches reveal little, don't be afraid to ask for librarian or study group facilitator assistance. Sometimes your adviser will know more appropriate key words for the search, or could introduce you to another collection (perhaps of research reports) that address your needs.
- If you are working with a colleague, establish clearly who is covering which aspects of the search. Avoid overlap or gaps between your investigative work.
- Make sure you have sufficient money/charge on your photocopy card to ensure that you can secure material that may need several readings.
- If you are making notes from texts within the library, always preface your notes with full details of the reference and its source (you may need to return to it again).
- Plan your library searches for times of the day when you are fresh and when library use by others might not be quite so heavy. It can be tedious and unproductive to spend a long time in the photocopy queue.
- Remember, libraries hold other media, e.g. audio and video tapes. Don't forget to consider such sources.

Where you look at documents not supplied through a library or from your own personal collection, it is important to recognize that they are someone's property. This is true for individuals (patients' case notes), organizations (a hospital cross-infection control policy) and for governments (e.g. policy documents published through the Department of Health, UK). Where documents have been published and are intended for use within the public domain, there are usually no problems about accessing these and making notes. Where, however, documents are in the private domain (i.e. not published or indicated for use by practitioners other than within restricted circumstances), it is necessary to seek permission before reviewing these. Patients in particular have a right to control who has access to their records, for purposes other than the delivery of treatment or care (McEnvoy, 1999; Pennels, 2001). Having obtained permission to review such documents, it will be necessary to manage this information with integrity and care. This extends to protecting the identity of individuals concerned, and to securing your records in a safe place so that they cannot be accessed by other individuals and for other purposes. For the document owner to give an informed consent to your request, you should provide a brief and clear explanation of your investigation and its purpose.

There is a wide range of documents that could prove useful. These include textbooks, journal articles, research papers or reports, policy statements, reflective diaries, the minutes of meetings and newspapers. In some extreme examples even artistic documents (e.g. a play script) might prove useful, were you to be investigating the treatment of a subject. At a local level, correspondence, requisition documents, budgets and similar might yield valuable information provided that you have proceeded in an ethical manner. If in doubt about accessing private documents, please check with your study group facilitator. He or she will assist you to judge the sensitivity of a document, who owns the document and what approach might be most appropriate if you wish to access it.

To ensure that documents serve your investigation, it will be important for you to read with a purpose. However interesting the material is, you should not forget that this is an information source to help you solve a problem or map a situation. You can keep your purpose in mind by writing key questions or aims down on a book marker that you use with your chosen documents, or by taking photocopies (where permitted) and using a highlighter pen to mark up only those passages that seem strictly important. Try to ensure that you highlight no more than 20 per cent within any one photocopy – a useful discipline that will help you achieve a clear focus.

You will need to content-code what you have read, in such a way that it can be succinctly reported back to your study group colleagues. There are a number of ways of coding documents but, simply put, they all refer to picking out the most important points from a work and then recording these in such a way that they have purchase upon your problem. Codes are short-hand expressions of more complex material within the original document. Each code should enable you to recall the point you want to explain to colleagues and include a specific reference, including page number for the source where you derived the code. In Table 5.2 I illustrate a code derived from short passages of text. This relates to an investigation associated with fertility cancer treatment (Foster, 2002). One article or typescript may yield several codes, each of which can be reconsidered in the light of subsequent reading.

Notice in this example how the code sums up a concern – at what point does infertility become permanent? This seems important because it informs the ways in which nurses respond to patients' questions – the way in which informed consent to treatment is obtained. The investigator does not stop there though, but goes on to record a couple of questions that can drive further reading and be offered to study group colleagues

Table 5.2   Coding from documents or interview transcripts

Source material	Code
The impact of chemotherapy drugs on sperm production in men is similar in many ways to the effect of radiation. Chemotherapy damages the rapidly dividing, ripening sperm cells. If damage is severe, the stem cells (mother cells) die as well. The higher the total dose of a damaging chemotherapy drug, the more slowly the recovery of sperm cell production, or the more likely it is to stop permanently.	*Permanent infertility* Questions: Are the critical chemotherapy doses likely to result in permanent infertility clearly known and communicated? Are there other factors that affect this? Are there margins of safety, between temporary and permanent infertility smaller with particular cytotoxic drugs- if so, which?

Source: Foster, R. (2002) Fertility issues in patients with cancer, *Cancer Nursing Practice*, 1(1), pp. 26–30 (p. 27)

later on. Questions such as these help the group to refine their understanding of a subject or problem, and may suggest new inquiries, perhaps in this case with a consultant or Clinical Nurse Specialist in oncology nursing. Within this example the original text is typed out in full. This is a good practice where the investigator senses that his or her coding might be more tentative. Where, however, you are confident that you understand what a text means, you may simply record the source, including relevant pages before writing down codes, associated questions or reflections.

Coding inherently involves a question – what does this mean? You will sometimes need to check this out with an investigative colleague, or to present a number of possible interpretations that the rest of the group can assist you with. It is important to acknowledge doubts at this stage because in fact, comprehension of health documents is not easy and it is quite possible to make mistakes based upon misconceptions from reading. Group facilitators spend time challenging such misconceptions. For this reason there is no shame in asking others' opinion on the nature or significance of information. By keeping an open mind and continuing to wonder what is happening here, you are likely to secure better information and to use it more wisely later on during collective analysis.

GATHERING INFORMATION FROM PRACTICE OBSERVATION

Contrary to what you might imagine, significant information can be gleaned from observation of and during practice and without the need for separate field trips where you act as the outside observer. What is important, however, is that your observations remain ethical, that you develop techniques to help you remain alert to observation opportunities and that you find a way of recording observations that enable you to share your new insights with others. Ethics first. Your observations are being planned as part of a modest inquiry, and will not usually be published. Like researchers, however, you are bound to observe in such a fashion that others' privacy is not gratuitously invaded, that respects their anxieties or concerns and which enables them to have some say in what is used for the problem- or enquiry-based group discussions ahead (Kennedy, 1999). In many instances observations will take place in your own practice environment, or during a clinical placement. It is often unnecessary to observe covertly. At the start of an investigation explain that your group is interested in a particular aspect of practice (e.g. risk assessment) and that you hope to use reflections upon this in practice to help inform group thinking. Asking colleagues (and patients or relatives if the observations focus upon interaction involving them) how they feel about your planned observations is an important first step and should be combined with a short briefing on your group interests. Once colleagues or clients have agreed to observations being made and recorded, it is then possible to proceed, making relevant notes that always identify the important stakeholders. In this way you can later check their comfort with any observations that you plan to debate within the study group.

Some of your observations are likely to be directed at how you practise and how you think. Reflection is an important part of nursing practice, and the more reflexive and quizzical about this you can be as part of your investigation, the better (Bolton, 2001). Even here, however, remember that your actions and communication impinge upon others whose permission might need to be sought before you can freely add your observations into the discussion pot.

Three techniques that appear to help observers remain sensitive to the investigation subject are set out in Box 5.2. What they have in common is that observers see the commonplace as strange, as something intrinsically worthy of asking questions about.

Box 5.2   Remaining alert to practice information

Quizzical questions

In this technique the observer identifies 2–3 questions that will be posed again and again during the shift. These may be written down as *aide-mémoires* but the very best ones are quite simple. For example, 'How do we respond to patient anxiety?' Questions are chosen because they are central to the investigation and likely to be answered in practice through a number of different episodes.

> ### What is the thinking behind this?
>
> The observer plans to observe a series of practices, usually those that are repeated, perhaps with different clients over the course of a shift. In each instance the investigator makes a mental note to observe the practitioner's actions intently and how the client or patient responds. Thereafter, the observer asks the practitioner a series of planned questions about how action here was connected to knowledge, beliefs and values.
>
> ### Alien visitor
>
> Rather more entertainingly the observer tries to imagine her or himself as an alien guest within the practice environment. Custom, the ways in which health care is interacted must necessarily be seen as something strange. The observer tries to identify the ways in which interaction is sustained – what, for instance, enables the patient to trust the practitioner in this setting?

Johns (2000) and Eraut (1990) have proposed a variety of reflective frameworks designed to make explicit the tacit knowledge used in practice. These are well worth examining, although individual nurses differ in what format of records they find most useful. Importantly such frameworks for reflection need to include not only an account of what happened during a particular clinical episode but also the following:

- Actions and reactions (nursing is concerned with communication, verbal and non-verbal and reactions to nursing actions can indicate something about the effectiveness or sensitivity of practice measures).
- Motives (what were you trying to achieve – were you clear about this?).
- Feelings (nursing involves emotional work, there is, for instance, stress associated with caring for dying patients or people dealing with chronic illness. Interaction with other health care professionals may also prove stressful. Of course other practice is particularly rewarding and it is worthwhile identifying exactly what makes a part of care delivery satisfying).

- Contexts (care episodes happen in a context, so it's often important to include details of what preceded an episode of care, what concerns stakeholders brought to it).
- Time frame (clinical episodes take on a clearer meaning when we understand the time frame involved. For example, client reactions may be influenced by the fact that they could 'sleep on' their treatment options).
- Location (the physical environment within which an episode takes place may also influence what was said and done).
- Consequences (what you think this means for your practice in the future, would you, for instance, change your approach next time?)

Unless you have the luxury of observing practice as a guest, with no other role, it's usually the case that you will need to make your observation records some time after the event. Memory can influence your account, so it is wise to make your records as soon as possible, either during a coffee break or straight after the shift. Even if you plan to write up fuller notes during the evening or the next day, it is worth making an outline of your impressions as quickly as possible. Creating an *aide-mémoire* will help you write up your observations accurately later on (see Figure 5.3).

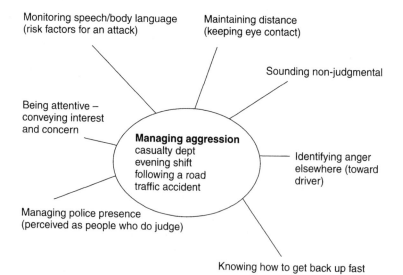

Figure 5.3   Example of an observation *aide-mémoire*

Aide-mémoires can take many forms, be jotted down in a pocket notebook or even recorded on a dictaphone if you prefer. Their purpose is simply to keep data fresh for when you can interpret it further.

One of the advantages of a diagramatic representation of an observation is that subsequently questions can be asked about how the different components fit together one with another. In this example, for instance, the investigator was particularly interested in how casualty department nurses manage the presence of police officers. The police needed to conduct their investigations and to interview patients, they provided an additional protection against possible aggression within the department. Against this, however, police officers were considered by many patients to ascribe blame, simply through their lines of inquiry. Patients felt vulnerable and ill prepared to respond clearly, or at least, in their own best interests. Nurses therefore had to manage the police presence so that patients were not provoked into aggression, some of which might be directed at the nurse. This was achieved by maintaining a treatment and support protocol first. Patients were protected from interview until they were appraised of their injuries after the accident. Notice in this example how the investigator makes a note of the context of the observation and the location where it occurred. Additional notes could have been added concerning whether the department was busy and what levels of practitioners were involved in managing the aggressive interlude. The *aide-mémoire* concentrates upon the nurses approach/handling of the situation. It could equally, however, have been focused upon the sequence of events and represented as a time line (see Figure 5.4).

GATHERING INFORMATION FROM FIELD TRIPS

Most of us have memories of completing field trips at school. They are frequently associated with the need to be well behaved and equally remembered for the embarrassment of the teacher when none of the pupils ventured a question afterwards. Field trips within PBL/EBL investigations need to be rather better organized and considerably more proactive. Goals for the field trip, questions that you hope to have answered, need to be set

Patient	Other parties
21.17 Patient swearing – accusing driver B of being drunk and reckless. Shouts over cubicle wall that B better watch out for himself	21.20 Nearby police officer steps in and cautions the patient not to be abusive. Policeman leaves cubicle.
	21.30 Attendant nurse enters with suture pack for cut to scalp. She is quizzed why she let the 'bloody cops in'.
21.35 Patient accuses the nurse of colluding with the system, assuming that he is in the wrong for this accident.Patient shoves the nurse to the floor and kicks her leg as he goes to leave.	21.40 The nurse stops the patient, assuring him that nothing has been assumed, if he had kept calm the policeman would not have stepped in. The policeman was there incidentally, associated with another accident.
21.45 Patient states he plans to take his own discharge and apologizes for 'tripping' over the nurse.	21.50 Nurse states his safety is paramount – he needs his wound tending. For now she decides not to call for back-up(situation retrieval)

Figure 5.4   *Aide-mémoire* (time line event)

down in advance. If the field trip requires access to be negotiated, it is polite to provide a letter setting out your aspirations for the trip, the questions that you hope to explore while on the visit.

In making a field trip visit it is important to consider a number of niceties if you are to gather the richest possible information. These include:

• Demonstrating respect for the work/approach of the team or organization that you visit (this may not be how you practise locally, but you are there to understand different ways of doing things).
• Being attentive (your set of questions represent your agenda, but remember too that your host may have an agenda of his or her own. Such visits might represent an opportunity for them to expound their philosophy. Field trips usually involve work on both agendas).
• Phrasing questions sensitively and timing them well (avoid posing potentially embarrassing or sensitive questions in front

of clients, for instance, and save more philosophical/approach questions until you have seen more of the operation. Additional silent observation may answer your question anyway).

- Providing a context or explanation for the focus of your question (you are trying to help the host answer as fully as possible. The more you share of your interest or motive, the more frank your host might be).
- Ensuring that you conclude your visit with thanks which should normally be expressed in writing after your return to base.

Field trips are useful ways of gathering new information in a variety of PBL/EBL circumstances. These are illustrated in the following quotes from students who employed them at various stages within an investigation:

> We were at the *what might be a better approach* in our project and sent three of our team to different units, all of which dealt with depressed patients in one guise or another. What we were after was not so much a plan for how things must be done as fresh ideas on what worked to a degree, given a certain sort of client circumstance. We got plenty of that and suggested three ways forward that could help our patients in the next year or so.
>
> (Eric, mental health care)

> When we went to visit the stoma care specialists at the district hospital it wasn't because we thought they could turn us into specialists overnight. It was because we wanted to find a clear boundary with them, to review when it was right to refer patient problems to them and when we could do something useful ourselves. Our problem was defining the boundaries and getting to know these people. In those terms, the visit helped because not only did we get more information but because we met people and got to know them.
>
> (Shona, primary practice nurse)

In the first example Eric and his colleagues pursue visits with a clear purpose – the expectations are realistic and met. These are visits comparatively late within an investigation when the problem has been deconstructed. It is conducted as part of the work towards solutions. In the second case, Shona is equally focused in the purpose of her visit. It is to get a stoma care specialist perspective on referral boundaries and upon relative expertize. The additional and unexpected benefit arises out of the fact that communication associated with the visit provides part of the solution, a more collegiate form of referral. Field trips are therefore useful to places of contrasting practice and where different perspectives upon or contributions to care need to be understood.

Making notes after such visits is an eclectic matter, but the golden rule remains, write up observations promptly and use a framework that makes sense to your group. This may simply be arranged as notes responding to a series of questions (printed in italics). It may also consist of field visit materials, for instance where you annotate another unit's philosophy of care, prospectus or patient education literature in order to highlight how they tackle problems. With your notes keep a copy of the host person's contact details (there may be other questions later on) as well as a copy of the thank you letter so that everyone knows that the etiquette of this information gathering is complete.

Conclusion

The most impressive and far-reaching PBL/EBL projects are founded upon well-organized and thoughtfully conducted information gathering. This is not only because you increase the array of data available for you to analyse but because you increase the range of contacts, the number of experts and other advisers who could potentially comment upon your project analysis. Learning to gather information in different ways, actively considering how you access information, the way you arrange interviews, how you make observations and record your thoughts are all skills that can be re-employed in this project and the one that comes beyond. While your interviewing, observing and reflecting have here been used in the service of a project, they are skills that can be employed to good effect in clinical practice. The more cognizant you are of how you used such questions, observations and notes, the better equipped you are to approach health care work in a conscious and effective way.

Having read this chapter you should have some fresh new ideas about conducting a PBL or EBL study. There are hints and good practice tips here that should make your information gathering more fruitful and stimulating. This is an important consideration, because the more enjoyable information gathering is, the more you will be motivated to press your project on. Good quality information stimulates debate and encourages you to think laterally about health care. The more ways you have found to think about a problem or need, the more flexible you will become in solving the problem or understanding the practice. In these terms, well-organized PBL/EBL information gathering can help accelerate the learning that you might otherwise accrue very slowly through clinical experience.

Gathering information can, however, be conducted in other ways, using the services of technology and the World Wide Web. It's to this additional source of information and inquiry that we now turn in the next chapter. As you read on remember, however, that no source of information is inherently superior to another. What is important is that you understand what the source *might* offer and what you hope to obtain there. Learning to select and access your sources wisely and cost effectively is an important part of practice development in health care.

6 USING THE INTERNET

At the close of the twentieth century nurse education entered a technological revolution which has the potential to transform the ways in which we obtain and use knowledge and which has significant benefit when problem- and enquiry-based learning is considered (Bramley, 2001; Johnson, 2001; Ward, 2001). The revolution centres upon the Internet or World Wide Web (an extensive and growing network of information sources spanning continents) and the computer/communication technology which enables investigators to access the different web sites, wherever these are located. Students studying first registration nursing today are already likely to be computer- and web-literate (at least regarding the gathering of information), while most learners may have used computers to word process documents, communicate by email and perhaps to 'surf' or shop for goods. In one recent survey of distance learners at the RCN Institute, the majority of students told us that they had access to a web-linked computer (either at work or at home), that they had used emails and visited websites. Some were, however, less confident about evaluating web information and communicating via the Internet. This chapter provides a basic introduction to gathering and sharing information using the Internet and assumes some rudimentary knowledge of computers. It cannot replace a whole programme on information technology, nor can it improve upon hands-on guidance in using a computer. It does, however, set out the principles of accessing web sites, evaluating information found there, downloading this and perhaps communicating findings and ideas to colleagues, typically by email.

WHAT IS THE WORLD WIDE WEB?

One of the simplest ways to describe the World Wide Web is with reference to an analogy. It consists of sources of information, located within servers, each of which has an address (an URL, Uniform Resource Locators), that can be accessed using a web-linked computer, using a modem and the telephone network of one or more countries. To help you search for relevant web sites you can employ a 'search engine' (e.g. yahoo) that tracks down relevant web sites using key words that you type into the computer. The web is rather like a town (but on a massive scale). Within our 'town' there are multiple addresses and of course various ways of finding your way around (signposts). Our town is within the 'Wild West'. That is, while the technology is well established and the means of getting from A to B are widely understood, what goes on within the town may not be regulated. Our town spreads across international borders so it is difficult to control. Web sites are rather like the businesses and residences within that town.

The reason why people have moved into the town are many and varied, but one thing is certain, their motives for being there are not solely to provide you with information. In some cases they have taken up residence to sell you a product or service (in which case the web address or URL often has the suffix .com, short for commercial). The web site address for the publishers of this textbook for instance is http://www.palgrave.com/home/ while that for a commercial supplier of stoma care equipment is http://www.convatec.com/. Such companies may share a certain amount of free information that could prove very useful, such as catalogues or advice about their products, but both Palgrave and Convatec are businesses. In other web sites the aim is to promote a cause, while for others it is more prosaically because individuals or groups wish to help others, sharing information freely and sensitively. Web site providers who provide a service to nurses, especially their members often suffix their web address with .org (short for organization). For example, http://www.rcn.org.uk will lead you to the Royal College of Nursing, while http://www.ino.ie/ will guide you to the Irish Nurses Organization, both of which provide excellent resources. Incidentally, the last suffix tells you within which country the organization is based, in this case the United Kingdom (uk) and the Republic of Ireland (ie) respectively. Web site providers who suffix their addresses with .edu (short for education) are usually universities or other institutes of learning. There you may find information about research, courses or conferences.

As in most other towns it is quite possible to get lost, or to visit places that won't meet your needs. What you are told in this town may not always be true, so it is important to check the source of your information. The World Wide Web is a fast

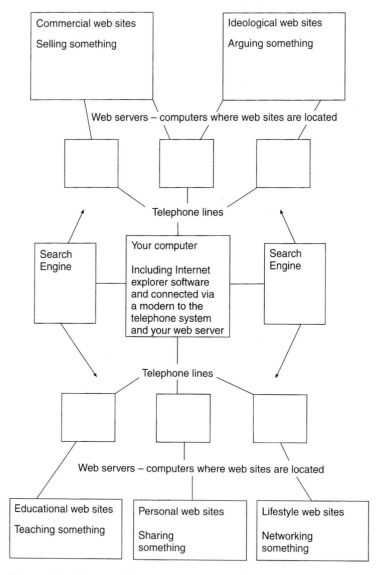

Figure 6.1   The World Wide Web

developing place so web sites come and go, and customs change. McCue (2002) commenting on the British Library's efforts to catalogue web sites observes that the average life span of a web site is just six weeks. Web sites that existed one month ago may no longer be there the next. To be fair, the more transient web sites are usually those set up by individuals or small groups, rather than large organizations. This said and returning to our Wild West analogy, towns that grow at this rate are not developed to a master plan. However tempting it might be to analogize the Internet to a massive library, this would be erroneous. It is not this organized, nor is it arranged so as to categorize information for you. When you enter this town you will make your own way, ask directions and decide what you buy, share or accept.

Rather simplistically the World Wide Web can be represented diagrammatically using boxes and lines (see Figure 6.1).

ACCESSING WEB SITES

We can explain how the web works with reference to example inquiries. In the first let's assume that you are studying within a university that has its own server. That is, it has a main frame computer with lots of memory capacity and a range of resources located within it. This might include electronic journals from which you can download articles, an alumni association where you can obtain details of other graduates and a comprehensive list of all the academic staff with their fields of expertize. By typing in the relevant access code for such services you can visit a number of these services by following the instructions that then appear on screen. You are using what is called the *intracom* or *intranet.* Your inquiries have probably never left the university or its campus, but you have quickly accessed information that would otherwise require significant fieldwork. Within the PBL/EBL context, for instance, that might include details of experts to interview, articles to read and university departments to visit.

Let's imagine, however, that what you seek (perhaps information on social science research) is not located within your particular university. This is not one of the disciplines served there. You have been advised that this information exists within particular web sites and have been given the address for these (e.g. http:// www.socresonline.org.uk – an online social research journal produced at the University of Surrey). Having opened the Internet access software within your computer, you type in the first address and this takes you via the modem and telephone line to the relevant server. Your inquiry travels via the telephone to the Internet server where you (or your employer) subscribes and from there by telephone line again to the web site in another server, possibly thousands of miles away. As you work, you are connected via this server by telephone line, incurring whatever charge exists associated with your own Internet server company, and possibly the cost of a local telephone call (package fees vary). As you open this web site you may be able to browse through several pages within the site by double clicking your computer mouse on the various icons. In the example above you can search for key terms such as 'ethnography', which will help you to identify relevant articles published on this subject. In some instances such clicking will connect you to not only different pages within this site but onward to other related web sites where more information exists. Your are now searching the *Internet*, the collection of web sites that in more or less tenuous ways serves a subject/topic or discipline. Because the web site addresses will change as you do this (see the web address window on your computer screen), it will be important to keep a note of these, either manually or by adding the address to your collection of 'favourites' using the tool bar on your computer screen.

Now let's imagine that you have a subject or question, but you do not have any target web sites that you would like to visit. At this stage you are unsure what these might be. You therefore open your computer and click on the web search engine included within the software package (for example, 'Yahoo'). Web search engines are commercial, located within large web servers that maintain large database searching facilities. They scan web sites connected by key words and offer them up within a menu of options. By clicking on the chosen title (itself an URL), you will be automatically connected to the appropriate web site. Some search engines focus upon web sites within a particular country or region (e.g. Europe) while others deal rather more globally. What they have in common is that they are only as helpful as the words that you key in for them to search. The search engine will pick out all literal connections to the word that you introduce, as some nurse students found to their surprise when they typed in 'rubber' while concluding a project on latex allergy. Were you to type in a term such as 'social research', for instance, it is likely that you would receive a large hit list of possible web sites, among them universities and their research departments, social science think tanks and or agencies that conduct surveys of public opinion. As with library catalogue searching, using such engines it is usually necessary to type in rather more discrete terms. For example, entering 'homelessness', or terms such as 'Shelter' (the name of a charity) is likely to prompt the suggestion of particular web sites, some of which may include research, policies or papers on the subject that you require.

Web sites are not formally categorized by type, although for practical purposes and as illustrated within Figure 6.1 you will see that we might usefully think of them in five terms. Many of the web sites you visit are likely to be composite, providing, for example, a certain amount of free information (example journal articles) but then promoting other products (the journal) as a purchasable product, either online (via the web) or as something mailed to your door (paper-based). In gathering information from the web it is important that you understand what sort of web site you are visiting and appreciate the constraints that this involves.

Commercial web sites

Commercial web site operators make their money either by charging you to view the contents of their site (through credit card payment), or by selling you a product having demonstrated to you the merits of what they offer through sample material. Such sites include journal publishers, many of which are switching their provision from paper to online-based services. You should not expect a commercial organization to provide liberal amounts of free information for download to your own computer. They may, however, provide incidental and useful examples of information, especially journal articles that could assist your inquiry. If you are seeking a comprehensive array of journal articles, it is much better to access a university library web site with its selection of electronic-based journals. If you are a university student, this service is often included with your programme registration fee.

Where commercial web sites may be more fruitful, however, is where you are investigating medical products and their use. Such sites may then provide extensive details of their own company products, access to a consumer adviser on using the product and perhaps details of regional representatives who might be able to tell you more about how the product is designed. Where a company wishes to promote its product it may publish research or product evaluation studies. Do be aware, however, that such sponsored research may be subject to bias.

Ideological web sites

Ideology has a part in most of our lives and there is nothing intrinsically wrong in accessing an ideological web site. These include those associated with political parties, with trade unions or pressure groups and sometimes even those associated with medicine or charities that include promoting a cause as part of their role. Professional bodies associated with nursing or medicine could be considered to provide ideological web sites (promoting the profession and arguing the merits of certain courses of action), but here the 'message' may be much subtle. Government web sites also offer a blend of policy and factual information, combined with a representation of health and health care as understood by the party in government.

Ideological web sites provide vivid illustration of polemical positions, stances upon health care and the needs or rights of specific stakeholders. They can illuminate the different ways in which a subject is understood. For instance, the UK National Health Service is understood rather differently by the various political parties, even if all subscribe to its merits in general terms. Visiting a political party web site gives you one perspective on the subject.

Educational web sites

Many web site designers claim to provide an educational web site and these include charities associated with health care (educating the public) and professional bodies such as the Royal College of Nursing or the Irish Nurses Organization. Those web sites that are solely committed to providing education are, however, much rarer on the World Wide Web and include publishers of Internet encyclopaedias such as *Encarta*. In some sites you are required to pay a subscription for access rights – something that individuals or families sometimes consider worthwhile when comparing this cost against the purchase of a large numbers of books. In the case of professional nursing organizations such as the Royal College of Nursing or the Irish Nurses Organization access to education (for instance, information from forums, or best practice guides) is often included free of charge, or subsidized by membership fees.

Personal web sites

The software packages now exist for individuals to create quite sophisticated web sites which they locate upon a web server and which might be identified through a search engine. In the majority of these cases the site contains family information, is lighthearted in nature or designed to help people with the same name network or trace their genealogy. Other such sites, however, may be used to promote the individual and his or her business or personal interests and can express extreme views or perspectives. Such web sites may be transitory upon the web, either because of the cost of maintaining them there, or because a web server company has refused to carry the site material after complaint.

These web sites have a very limited value in PBL/EBL inquiry but they may occasionally provide personal testimony regarding a health care problem. For instance, some personal web sites might describe the handling of chronic illness, dealing with health care bureaucracy or promote coping strategies that have worked for this individual. It is highly eclectic information but may illustrate aspects of a problem under investigation. The sites are usually found via web search engines when you use an illness term that the individual has included among key words describing his or her site, when hiring space on the web server.

Lifestyle web sites

Here the term lifestyle web sites describe those which espouse particular practices, beliefs or values, some of which may be unusual or even abhorrent to the investigator. Such web sites need to be approached with extreme caution, both because the views expressed within them could seem distasteful and because regularly connecting to them may in some instances leave you open to criminal investigation. Pornography and paedophilia, for instance, do exist on a number of web sites. As was indicated earlier within this chapter, the World Wide Web is not regulated to the degree that information services are elsewhere. Within the web there exist extreme perspectives that are uncomfortable to examine.

You may wonder why an investigator would wish to visit any such site. In practice, some are happened upon by chance (while surfing the web) while others are targeted as part of a legitimate investigation. Consider, for instance, a project that examines health promotion and risk-taking behaviour associated with sexually transmitted diseases. In such an investigation it may be relevant to understand how others see risk and manage this as part of a lifestyle. Clients lead different lives and have different values. Under these circumstances it could be important to learn about alternative values and practices expressed within a web site (for instance regarding 'swinging' – the swapping of sexual partners).

Having found useful web sites and material within them, it is important to prepare a reference that enables you and other group members to find the resource again. It is important to include the date when you accessed the web site, so that others are warned that the material may have subsequently changed, or the web site might have disappeared completely. Copy down all reference details with great care as the various digits and symbols of the address may be case-sensitive and spacing and stop marks are just as important as letters or numbers. Here is an example of web address referencing: 'http://www.ino.ie/ Web site of the Irish Nurses Organization, accessed 29 April 2002'. This very simple reference simply alerts your colleagues to the existence of a web site and who runs it. The title by itself, ino might not otherwise immediately alert them that this site is provided by the Irish Nurses Organization.

If you have found a specific resource within a web site, however, you will need something rather more detailed. Here the conventions of paper-based referencing are still followed but with additional detail that guides the reader to the source. For example, here is a reference to an online article.

Finlay, A. (1999) '"Whatever you say say nothing": an ethnographic encounter in Northern Ireland and its sequels', *Sociological Research Online*, 4 (3), socresonline/4/3/finlay.html> (accessed 29 April 2002)

The reference provides detail of the author and date of publication first. This is followed by the title of the article and the journal where it is located. There is the usual volume number and then the issue number, in brackets. Page numbers are replaced by the URL contact details. Notice the phrase html> at the end. This signifies the sort of text the article has been prepared within.

EVALUATING WEBSITE INFORMATION

Web information comes in many different forms and you may require specialist programmes to decipher some of this (e.g. Acrobat Reader). Web sites are composed of text and pictures, they may include video clips or sound, so simple word programmes will not always serve your purpose. This said, many of the appropriate software files can themselves be downloaded from the Internet, and within a web site you may see an icon that you can click on to do just that.

This acknowledged, whatever you access there is still a need to evaluate the merits of such material. The above typology of web sites suggests that it is important to understand what sort of information you are reading and to understand just who has posted this. In Box 6.1 I suggest a number of useful questions that you might ask of information that you view on web sites.

Box 6.1   Questions to ask when visiting a web site

- What type of web site is this, does it address the subject matter I thought it did and do I wish to explore here?
- Which organization or individual runs this web site and therefore plays editor to what is included there? Are there any biases here?
- Is the site well organized and laid out? A very sophisticated site does not automatically contain useful information, but it suggests that the site may well still be there tomorrow. Your group colleagues may need to visit the web site later on.
- When I click on icons to access useful information, do I remain within this web site or get directed to a completely

---

Box 6.1   (*continued*)

different one (a frame will come up warning you that you are being redirected to a new web site by such hypertext links)? It is important at this stage to again review the new web site address, its type and to question just who runs it. Within a web surfing session its relatively easy to change web sites in this way without realizing that you are dealing with several different organizations.

- Who posted the information and when? Where web-based research or other papers are published, a quality site will normally require that the posting date be shown. This enables you to judge how old the work is, either by such details being added to the top of the page or because the material is arranged in 'year/issue volumes' much like a paper-based journals.

- What is your impression of the scholarship of the material written there? For instance, is there reference to the literature and is a reference list/bibliography included? Is the tone academic or colloquial? Does the material appeal to research, anecdote or product evaluations? Search for clues that the work is considered and authoritative. You may feel encouraged if the work included the opportunity to email the author through a hypertext link. In this way you can verify further the claims being made or perhaps extend your investigation with the expert.

- What was the context of the work being presented in this site? If this isn't stated, it is worth looking for signs that it has simply been transported onto the site from a previous and possibly paper-based publication. You can sometimes sense this when the work doesn't make use of devices within the site to enhance illustration. In most instances such transportation of papers into a site is quite legal and arranged by a publisher. Sometimes work (even novels) are written for dissemination on the Internet. In a few rogue cases, however, the work may have been plagiarized or posted on the site without the author's knowledge. In these instances you may need to question the authority of what is written there.

DOWNLOADING INFORMATION

Having found a rich resource on the web, the next question is whether to print off a copy of what you see or to download the various files and store them on your computer. Beware of downloading files unless you have an up-to-date virus protection software loaded on your computer. One or more files may contain a virus that could destroy a lot of the information you have already gathered, be transmitted to the computers of other group members as well as damage other files you have in your system. Once you have bought virus protection software and loaded it on your computer, arrange to take the updated versions as these become available, themselves as download files from the virus-checking software company.

In practice, some documents obtained via the Internet are quite extensive, particularly government papers or policy documents for instance. They become tiring to read on screen and there is then merit in arranging a print-out of the most important parts. If you print out the whole document you can then highlight that which you will cut and paste as most salient elements for discussion. Many web site documents include an 'executive summary', which might be sufficient for your purposes and can be downloaded or printed as a separate file.

By going to the file menu of your computer while the web site screen is open you are offered the opportunity to download one or more of the documents. You will be asked where you wish to save this material (which directory or folder within your system) and when the download is complete, the file will appear in your computer menu, detailing the nature of data contained within it. You provide the file title, but the computer will warn you whether it is, for instance, a photo file (e.g. Jpeg(fine) requiring specific software to open). Downloading of large amounts or complex format material can take some time, so plan when you will download information so that you can monitor progress and control costs.

COMMUNICATING USING INFORMATION TECHNOLOGY

Having considered information technology as a potential source of information, it is useful to consider also just how technology

---

Box 6.2   Communicating using technology

- Teleconference (using the telephone system, booked with a telephone service provider for a specific time and date, for a particular duration, and with a list of telephone numbers to be included within the conference.)
- Videoconference (this also makes use of the telephone network, but requires that group members have access to a video conferencing pack and web cam cameras before their image can be broadcast. Most video conferencing is conducted between institutional study centres.)
- Asynchronous conference boards (provided within a web site and permitting messages to be posted that other group members can add to. In this approach the group members are logged on to the web site at different times convenient to them.)
- CHAT Room networking (this also uses a web site conference system but the communication is synchronous or virtually synchronous. Typically group members type in their messages and the software orders the appearance of these in dialogue sequence or 'strings'.)

---

may be used to communicate what you have found out. PBL or EBL study groups are not necessarily located in one place. Group members may be scattered across a country, a continent or even the whole world. Within distance learning programmes, for instance, students may exist in several different countries and still keep in touch with their tutor who is UK-based. There are several different ways in which the group might communicate and these are set out in Box 6.2.

Teleconferences have a number of advantages where group member travel would otherwise prove prohibitive. To get the best from such an approach, however, it is important to have an agreed agenda for the meeting and a chairperson who will manage the discourse. A skilful chairperson will make sure that all group members are welcomed to the session, indicate when particular contributions are sought and ensure that no teleconferenced group member is left silent and isolated for too long. This is important for as discussion becomes more voluble, it is difficult to know when best to interject. You don't have faces around the table to assess concerning when an idea or suggestion would seem most welcome.

If there are papers to be read before the teleconference, it is important to email or mail these well in advance. Teleconference members need to be clear which paper they are referring to and with this in mind all papers should include page and section numbering. It makes good sense to ensure that the chair signals clearly when items are being left behind and what agreed action is to take place. At the end of the teleconference it is then helpful to prepare an action plan of what is being done next and by whom, within a particular time frame.

Videoconferencing works well within larger-scale projects where different groups, for instance in research, are connected to each other to discuss project progression or interim findings. It is, however, a relatively costly and sophisticated operation, not widely employed within problem- or enquiry-based learning. Rather more practicable may be the use of webcams (web cameras) attached to computers that enable group members to show colleagues visual information or objects that they have collected and which is not readily transmittable as a scanned image. While web cams have often been used socially, for instance, helping families keep in touch, there is little reason why they could not be used in the service of a problem- or enquiry-based learning group, provided that members recognized the definition of image limitations of such technology.

Asynchronous and synchronous (CHAT) conference boards, located and read through a web site involve a number of challenges. They consist of a visual series of entries from group members, indicating who posted the information and what he or she said (Stratfold, 1998). You post your ideas, comments, reflections and responses by typing these into a keyboard and submitting them as text to the web site. Very quickly the new contribution appears on screen, under a topic heading, for others to read either immediately, or later on at their leisure. It is often hard for individuals to type as fast as they can think and to relax concerning the submission of ideas in text form. We associate written documents or submissions with academic papers, something serious or perhaps weighty. When they appear on screen, our comments can seem very visible and permanent, compared with a conversation in the coffee room. Within conferencing, however, the hoped-for analogy is more to do with speech and debate, with individuals encouraged to type what they think, making suggestions or arguing a case as appropriate (Vincent and Whalley, 1998). Within any conversation about the problem or inquiry it is possible for a number strands of debate to develop. For example, a discussion about assessing mentally ill people may include strands on medical labels/professional power/tact/ethical practice and making records, each with a series of contributions made by group members. Because of this, group members need to be disciplined, indicating clearly to what they refer when they post a new offering. This is a considerable challenge when the dialogue between three or more group members become longer and longer, forming a string of information.

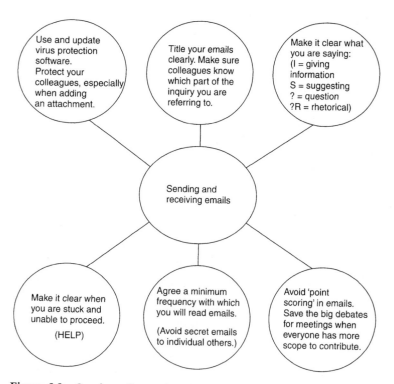

Figure 6.2   Good email practice within the study group

Such technology-based communication systems are liberating for groups that have membership spanning great distances (Eastmond, 1995; Jones, 1998). It is, however, worth remembering that the simplest forms of communication are usually the most sustainable. Where a physical meeting cannot be arranged, sharing information by email can be extremely effective (Edwards and Hammond, 1998). A simple email code of good practice will enable the group to keep successfully in touch between meetings (see Figure 6.2).

We have become used to seeing emails as short-hand and even colloquial forms of communication. 'Hi' replaces 'Dear Susan' and this works well within PBL/EBL group work. Do, however, bear in mind that the reader of your emails cannot see your facial expression. If you have a lot to communicate, it is still worthwhile coding the information so that the others know when you are informing them of something discovered, requesting help, being rhetorical or asking a question that you hope one or more of them will reply to. There is no standard abbreviation for such work so each group should feel free to develop their own. If these prove successful, they may be used again and again over several inquiries, speeding up the work completed and helping group members to get the most from problem-solving together.

CONCLUSION

The World Wide Web or Internet offers a range of additional information to the PBL/EBL study group and the means in some circumstances to compare notes about what has been discovered. Developments within information technology mean that groups do not have to work in the same geographical location. It is possible for problems to be analysed in several different hospitals, thousands of miles apart. The only limits to this are the imagination and technological skills of the group members.

This said, the Internet is not a panacea. Information found here might not be as authoritative as that found more conventionally within a library or through local fieldwork. It is important to understand the types of web sites from which information comes and to evaluate that information carefully, searching for bias. Because web-based information comes from many different organizations and people with different motives, it is necessary to be cautious when incorporating it within problem analysis or inquiry development. However exciting it may seem, it has been gleaned (at least beyond electronic journals and library web sites) from the Wild West end of the information spectrum. What appears upon a web site may have been vetted by the web server owners, but no claims are made as to the authority of the information there. The checks that are run usually focus upon whether the information is defamatory or likely to leave the web server owner open to prosecution. It is worth remembering that in most instances there is no professional librarian within the web, cataloguing and annotating the information that is daily added to the resource.

This chapter necessarily assumes a minimum amount of knowledge concerning accessing the web through a computer and modem. Its focus has been upon understanding the web as a source of information that might assist the study group. If you are not already familiar with web surfing (at least for educational purposes), I hope that it has alerted you to the web's potential and its limitations. It is well worth correcting any shortfall of information of skill concerning technology as part of PBL/EBL work. Not only will an 'Introduction to the web' short course at college increase the resources available to you, it can significantly reduce the amount of time and effort needed to pursue a particular investigation.

7 ANALYSING YOUR INFORMATION

Having now considered the different ways in which you may gather information, it is time to think about the analysis of what you collect. The process of analysis shapes raw information either towards a problem solution (PBL) or towards a fuller explanation of practice (EBL). While the goals of problem- and enquiry-based learning are different, most of the analysis measures are quite similar. There is a need to appreciate what information is before you, to judge whether this seems complete, coherent, clear or confusing, and to consider how the various bits of information might fit together. As with a jigsaw there is a need to test pieces of information to see whether they fit the picture. Intriguingly of course, this jigsaw does not have a picture to work from in the first place. In Chapter 2 (Figure 2.4) the components of problem analysis were described in terms of facts, learning issues, new inquiries and working solutions. The equivalent with enquiry-based learning would still include facts, learning issues and new inquiries, but working solutions are replaced by tentative explanations. Within EBL and PBL analysis the context of the investigation is usually important. Because practice demands vary according to context, and human beings are diverse in their requirements, analysis needs to take account of the context of the situation (see Table 7.1).

Analysis involves a number of related processes with which your study group should be familiar. These processes are designed to help you decide when, for the purposes of the project, information is counted authoritative enough to represent a 'fact'. They also help explain just why other information or interpretations remain within the learning issues box and prompt ideas about what additional inquiries still need to be made. Towards the end of a project they help the group sense when a satisfactory closure can be reached, and a problem solution recommended or an enquiry report prepared.

Table 7.1   Context and analysis

PBL study	EBL study	Contextual influences
Finding more persuasive ways of promoting breast-feeding among first-time mothers		The semi-public environment on the post-natal ward where breast-feeding success (or otherwise) might be judged
	Exploring the decision-making process associated with feeding during the last stages of terminal illness	Understanding the temporal dimension, how long will someone live, how near death are they? There is a need to assess when feeding supports physical comfort (e.g. reducing risk of pressure problems versus when it becomes unnecessarily intrusive in the last hours of life)

IDENTIFYING 'FACTS'

Agreeing what represents a fact in an investigation can be very difficult. Group members can and do appeal to different criteria regarding what represents the truth. For some this is seen in absolute terms. The fact must hold good in many different circumstances. It becomes akin to a scientific law, robust enough to predict what will happen within the future. For others a circumstantial fact might be accepted, provided that caveats remain about its use in other situations. Facts are, however, derived from collecting and relating information and interpreting what this collectively means. Because much nursing care deals with untidy social circumstances, and has to incorporate stakeholder perceptions, it is important to appreciate and respect the different ways in which perceptions of information are built up (see Chapter 1 for an account of the nature of problems).

In practice, however, study groups are forced to find ways of agreeing what counts as 'facts'. You will need to develop criteria by which you feel able to set aside certain information/interpretations as a given and to move on to another layer or part of the analysis.

This is important because in some projects the next part of your work assumes your previous agreement about certain facts. For instance, in the above problem analysis concerning breast-feeding, the group would have to agree that the benefits of breast-feeding, to baby and mother, are a fact. While there are inconveniences and discomforts associated with breast-feeding, on balance, the arguments in favour of breast-feeding outweigh the problems. Only by agreeing such facts does the group have the moral backing to consider ways of persuading a client to behave in a particular way. Practice must be based upon the principle of beneficence and challenges us to answer the question, 'Who knows best?' (Gillon, 1994).

Researchers and research teachers have spent a considerable time developing and debating what counts as fact or authoritative research evidence. Historically this consisted of asking whether data was valid, reliable and ethical (Hek, 1996). More recently writers have begun to recognize that such criteria betray a particular perspective on the world, what counts as the most important knowledge and what represents science. Positivists value knowledge that can be replicated in different contexts, study designs that can be repeated and researchers who adopt a dispassionate stance towards gathering and analysing the data. Factual knowledge consists of empirical data (i.e. that which can be observed and measured) combined with consistent and rigorous analysis methods (e.g. measurement instruments designed to capture data on a carefully defined phenomenon) (Lobiondo-Wood, 2002).

There are, however, other evaluative criteria used within research, and these often focus upon the authenticity of data. Such criteria are employed by researchers who work within the naturalist or critical theory paradigms, where research is conducted in the social world and where there is scant chance of the researcher controlling all the variables that might affect the results. This sort of research is evaluated in terms of whether there is a clear audit trail of how results were arrived at, and whether the resultant information sounds as though it fits in with your experience of the phenomenon in question (Koch, 1994). What is important about all of this is that evidence is evaluated with reference not only to the data itself, but to the stated intentions of the researchers, their design assumptions and philosophical premises. We pause and recognize what assumptions we hold

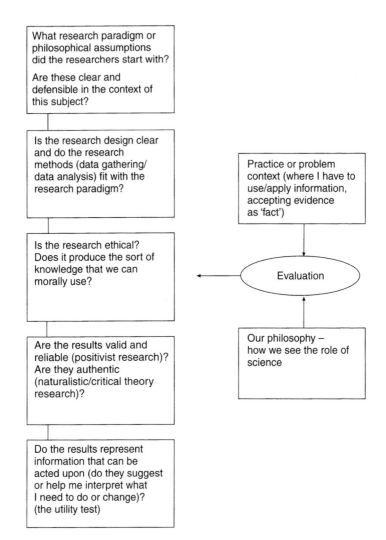

Figure 7.1 Evaluating research evidence

about science and knowledge as consumers of the research reports (see Figure 7.1).

Imagine that you are evaluating research evidence as part of your analysis. Whether or not this evidence counts as fact depends upon the extent to which the study answers your questions at each of the levels outlined in Figure 7.1. If the study is unclear in terms of underlying research paradigm or philosophy, it is difficult to ascertain what the researchers are claiming regarding the nature of truth. Very large textbooks are written on research design and evaluation, but briefly here, positivist design research presents research work as the search for a truth that can be observed and discovered again through a replicated study. These studies emphasize observation and measurement, the definition of key terms early on within the study design and careful structuring of the research so as to examine only the phenomena in question. To this end the researcher tries to minimize his or her influence upon the data, limiting bias in results (Weir *et al.*, 1999). Typically research is designed as a randomized control trial, an experiment or perhaps a descriptive survey with carefully worded questionnaire. Naturalistic paradigm research focuses upon the search for meanings within the health care world, accepting that there is no fundamental truth, only a series of interpretations or constructions of experience that individuals or groups create (Smith and Price, 1996). These researchers typically design their research using interviews, field observations and case studies, and invite participants to report their experiences and understandings. The data emerging from such studies are usually qualitative rather than quantitative. Critical theory paradigm research also focuses upon research within the natural environment, but in this instance the researcher acknowledges a philosophical perspective (perhaps feminist or Marxist). Such researchers question whether science can remain separate from politics and the commitment to better the lot of disadvantaged groups (Smith and Price, 1996).

There are several ways in which research design might fail to produce evidence that you can feel confident about. These include where the researcher states that the project was designed to help us understand the experience of others, but then makes recommendations about practice. At best, such a study can illuminate experiences and suggest what we need to consider during practice. Studies that report the experience of others are ill-placed to support specific actions. In this instance there is a poor fit between the design of the research (which set out to do one thing) and what the researcher claims on the basis of the data. Researchers need to avoid over-stating what the evidence can support, or alternatively, selecting research designs that cannot reasonably produce the sorts of data upon which recommendations can be founded.

If you are conducting problem-based learning as part of a course, you should turn to your taught sessions upon research and research evaluation to assist you with analysis. Alternatively, if you have not studied research at this stage it is important to ask your facilitator for assistance in judging the merits of information. If you are conducting an EBL project outside a course of studies, then it may be appropriate to consult a researcher or nurse teacher as part of your analysis. Either way, for you to incorporate research evidence within your work, you will need to appreciate the criteria used for its evaluation and to apply these thoughtfully to the research papers that come before you (see Figure 7.2). Don't guess the merits of research evidence. In the parlance of popular television quiz shows, 'phone a friend' and/or consult a text through which you can both evaluate the merits of the work (Polit, 2001).

It would be encouraging if the majority of information used within analysis was based on research evidence. In practice, the majority of information does not originate from research. It comes from your observations, interviews, reflections and the reading of articles, theories or clinical practice episodes. What criteria can be agreed here in order to decide what can be counted as at least a project fact? Evaluative criteria in this situation are necessarily softer than those used in research evaluation. They need to be worked through with fellow group members and your group facilitator, as part of what can be called 'rhetoric'. Dictionaries define rhetoric as the art of speaking or writing well or effectively. The term rhetoric has its origins in the first Greek democracies of the ancient world and refers to a process where peers debated the nature of truth and what could be relied upon as a basis for moral action. If you wish to learn more about rhetoric in these terms it is well worth reading Plato's *The Republic* which reports the arguments debated by philosophers such as Socrates (Plato, 1974). For our purposes, problem- and enquiry-based analysis requires you to develop the skills of rhetoric. That is, considering whether the information you hear seems true, whether it applies in the current context and whether there are any conditions or factors that might challenge this. Are there counter-explanations for what has been reported or seen? Are there more important information to be considered or given priority in this analysis? A skilful study group facilitator will encourage you to ask questions of your colleagues, to posit alternative explanations or ideas and

Positivist research
(e.g. experiments/randomized control trials/descriptive surveys with pre-set questions)

Validity: Is this data valid, reflecting what was observed/collected and representative of a wider population of people from which the sample was drawn?

Reliable: If this study was repeated, does it seem likely that very similar results would be obtained?

Naturalistic research
(e.g. grounded theory/phenomenology/ ethnography/case studies, open questionnaire surveys)

Authenticity: Judging by the audit trail, the account of how data was gathered and analysed, are these results likely to represent what participants said/shared?

Fit: Given that my local clients/patients/circumstances are very similar to those described in the study, have I witnessed similar results locally in practice?

Steps

1. Identify the research paradigm
2. Select the evaluative criteria
3. Judge the evidence
4. Check the ethics of the study
5. Consider how closely the evidence fits with your project context

Critical theory research
(e.g. action research, feminist phenomenology or ethnography, some forms of case study with a stated 'cause')

Authenticity: Critical theorists appeal to authenticity of their work on similar grounds as naturalist researchers above

Justice: Does the research attend to a social injustice, focus upon a need or problem and suggest insights or change that are defensible in terms of improving the lot of others?

Figure 7.2   Evaluative criteria for research evidence

to explore your values and beliefs. Remember, this is not combative. You are not trying to beat your colleague. Instead, the debate exists only in order to arrive at better explanations, better solutions. Sometimes these may be yours, but more often than not, they are a composite of several points, yours and others! Now let's look at some evaluative criteria and illustrate each as we go along.

What is being claimed?

It is important to be certain about what is being claimed as 'fact' within our project. Take a look at the following assertion made by a group member involved in an EBL project on patient self-medication in hospital. The group is interested in what would be involved if patients had control of their own medications within the ward environment:

> For us to support a self-administration policy you not only have to pro-vide secure storage of drugs in patients' lockers, you have to assess whether the patient and others are responsible enough to manage drugs in this way in a communal setting. My interviews suggest that staff were anxious about this because they're unsure whether patients will keep cupboards secure and whether other patients will resist the temptation to take drugs. However attractive it sounds, there is an elem-ent of trust involved here and meantime the hospital retains liability.

While this is only one short report of findings, several things are claimed. First, that patients might be forgetful or negligent in terms of securing medications, second, that some other patients could prove unscrupulous and steal drugs and, third, that staff are anxious about superintending such a system. I think that this colleague is clear about these claims, and that this is backed up with interview evidence. What may be less clear is whether some-thing is also being said about the motives for self-medication policies. Notice the remark 'about however attractive it sounds'. This could mean that this colleague is concerned about the motives behind such policies. Are they there for cost saving devices – to reduce the time spent by scarce staff on drug rounds? Before these points could be admitted as fact within this project it would be necessary for points such as this to be clarified. 'Do you think that the self-administration policy then is driven by cost-saving agendas? Is this wise with regard to the staff code of conduct?'

Is there sufficient evidence to support the claim?

Sometimes a claim is supported as fact because there is an over-whelming volume of evidence to suggest that this is true. It happens again and again and is reported by different people. Look at this example, where a group chair is summing up information provided by several of the group members about what worries parents about vaccinations:

> We seem to have this told to us from several angles. There's the parents Joyce has talked to in the clinic, there's the GP accounts we saw on the video and the material that keeps coming through in the literature that Steph summarized for us. Parents associate problems that arise about the same time as inoculations as being caused by the vaccin-ation. They assume that there are unrecognized interactions between components within a compound vaccination and that scientists are not being truthful. They base some of this on 'cover-up conspiracy' assuming that there is a percentage risk involved, but that governments want parents to take this risk, because the alternative is even more problematic.

Incidentally, this is a good example of chair summary in problem-based learning, but it also provides an opportunity to wonder if we have the whole story. We know what it is argued the parents fear, but do we have a representative picture of all that they think? Did Joyce ask parents who accepted a vaccination as well as those who refused? If not, these parents might have offered other ways of debating whether or not to proceed with vaccin-ations. While this may have included the ways they overcome their fears, it might also have suggested additional concerns that the first group did not recognize.

It is easy to conclude that there is never enough evidence to support a claim as fact and never enough time to gather more evidence. In these circumstances it is necessary to make a decision based upon the balance of evidence. The claim is then accepted as likely to be true, but marked with an asterisk, in case that subsequent evidence brings it back into question. In the above example patient fears (as reported) were considered likely to be accurate, but it was acknowledged that they might work with other personal factors such as their own family history of vaccin-ation uptake and experiences. Family folk wisdom might be as influential as whether parents trusted governments and scientists.

What other claims exist?

In many instances you might need to consider multiple and sometimes counter-claims about information available. This is particularly true within problem-based learning and often in association with the diagnosis of a patient's circumstances, signs or symptoms. Under these circumstances each of the claims has to be reviewed in terms of available supporting evidence and clarity of claim. Consider the situation where a study group was presented with the details of a 12-year-old boy who was behaving strangely within class. He seemed 'vacant' and inattentive. In the scenario supplied reference was made to a past road traffic accident and concussion, but there is also discussion of a 'glue sniffing' problem at the school. Here two Icelandic nurses debate what needs to be sorted out in evaluating competing claims:

> *Sigrun*: If this is epilepsy then we need a good history of how long it has been going on and whether it seems to have started after his accident. I'm not sure that these forms of epilepsy always come from trauma. He might have a tumour, or perhaps it has been there much longer and we can't find a cause.

> *Christian*: I think that's right. But we could discard the glue theory with some simpler investigations first. We could ask his mother whether she has seen any signs of soreness around his mouth or nose. There may be plastic bags, aerosols left lying around with the stuff in. She might also notice that his problems come in quick episodes, for instance, after he has been somewhere private for a while.

This is an exercise in 'differential diagnosis' but what is most important is that the group members are considering the conditions under which claims of fact can be accepted. Sigrun starts to map the health history that would need to be taken before the problem could be called epilepsy and linked to a particular cause. Christian suggests rather simpler, quicker assessments that might be employed to exclude the alternative diagnosis – to dismiss the claim that the boy's problems stem from substance abuse. These nurses have begun to consider not only what evaluative criteria might be employed here, but to appreciate what could be done first.

If this were true, what would be the consequence?

Sometimes claims are made for which there is insufficient evidence currently available but which the group is inclined to think may be true. Members take the view that the evidence has not yet formed. Under these circumstances they may decide to plan a number of speculative tests that will help them make up their minds. Within health care it is clearly inappropriate to experiment upon clients or colleagues, but it may be possible to plan observations of what happens naturally, so that cause and effect relationships, or significant correlations of behaviour can be investigated. In these circumstances the group members try to imagine what would happen if the claim were true? In the following example which concerns patients suffering from cancer and that which promotes treatment compliance, notice how these nurses establish what they agree would constitute proof of the claim:

Gemma: So if a relative, especially a partner, encouraged them to stick with the chemotherapy and we heard the patient talk positively afterwards about seeing the treatment through, that would count wouldn't it?

Annette: I think they would have to say that it was because so and so was wishing them on. Other things could be important to their motivation, so you'd need to make the link.

Gemma: I think it would have to last too. Their relative would have to be an influence when they were feeling poorly or fed up. You know, when they're feeling nauseated and you might expect them to think of giving up.

Annette: Yes... it's easy enough to notice these things too. Patients talk about what keeps them going all the time. We don't need to quiz them about this, just notice it when it happens.

It is as this point in analysis that connections are readily made between the evaluation of information, what counts as facts and where or how the group might make new inquiries. In this instance, additional observations within practice are planned. These will not only help the nurses check whether it is a fact that patients' partners are a significant support in motivation towards treatment but help them explore whether others factors (for instance, fear of relapse) are more significant.

Exploring learning issues

Making new inquiries and reaching solutions or conclusions are addressed within the next chapter, so now we will focus upon the remaining part of analysis – exploring the learning issues. For many group facilitators this is the most exciting part of the problem- or enquiry-based learning. It affords the opportunity for you to develop transferable skills and to appreciate just why you know something. Facilitators are excited by the prospect of helping you to understand how you think and what can be done to increase reasoning success in different situations. Students, however, sometimes think of the exploration of learning issues as more peripheral. It is uncomfortable enough to carry some debates as temporarily unresolved without also pausing to think about how they are using information. It is easy to become focused upon the pursuit of an answer, a solution to a problem or an explanation of practice, and to forget the signposts that enabled you to get there. However, if the techniques that you learned this time are to have beneficial effect in later projects, it is essential that you find time within your group work to consider learning issues.

Group analysis of problems or practice involves understanding how we have learned, what has and hasn't expanded our horizons. The first of these concerns the selection of different information, placing this side by side in some form of relationship in order to make sense of what has been gathered. Deciding what examples of information to relate to another is an important process because it helps us manage the analysis of the problem. The more you understand this, in terms of what you did, why you did it, and what pay-off it offered, the better able you will be to use the technique again.

Interrelating different information

To make this point clear let's consider an example which stems from a problem-based learning project on working with relatives. In this case study students were given a scenario where an elderly man is admitted to hospital and the patient's daughter demands to speak to the senior nurse of the ward. She is angry about the delay in finding her father a bed and now demands to know what the ward nurses will do to assist him. In the scenario questions are posed about why the daughter is upset, what might be done to meet her needs and what this could mean for the future working relationship between professional and lay carer (the daughter). The nurses in this PBL group used the scaffold (described in Chapter 4) to help them unpick this situation and decide how to proceed if they faced the angry daughter. Discussion focused especially upon the frames of reference (how *should* the nurse relate to relatives? – how *should* relatives work with professional staff?) and the decision-making process. In this case the decision-making debates centred upon deciding how to 'think on your feet'. This was a relative who was angry and the nurse is taken unawares by her request.

The group were advised to review the frames of reference that nurses held for themselves and those they ascribed to others (lay carers). These were summarized on a flip chart before circumstantial factors, which the group believed would in some way influence whether the frame of reference could hold good, were added (see Figure 7.3).

The students conducted their decision-making analysis in terms of three principles: demonstrating respect and concern for the relative; being collegiate (not dumping a problem on a colleague); and norm setting (establishing a relationship which would be mutually respectful and sustainable over time). The students were then challenged with the question, 'What happens to the frames of reference when you're faced with a angry relative?' In this example the group agreed that normal frames of reference were suspended, at least, those that were ascribed to others. Faced with such a situation it was difficult to work out exactly what frame of reference the relative was working with. It was also questionable whether our previous assumptions about how others were behaving or would behave were accurate in the first place. Instead of seeing the relative as a potential resource with his or her own wisdom, relatives had to be seen in terms of additional casualties. We began a second round of discussion about relatives as casualties or carers and this emphasized the need to accurately assess what relatives needed first. In this acute situation the nurse was forced to listen very attentively and to demonstrate no obvious assumptions about lay carer responsibilities. We debated if this careful (and quite draining) assessment of the situation was required in this confrontation, what was it

Nurses	Relatives
Should brief relatives, subject to patient approval	Should respect the expertize of professionals
Should appreciate relatives' worry	Should recognize the need to prioritize care (the needs of all)
Should recognize relatives' expertize (experience of patient and his/her history)	Should try to work with the staff (e.g. supply relevant information)
Should try to involve relatives' in care (rehabilitation especially)	Should want to contribute to care (learn about the situation)
Should recognize relatives' limitations and/or capacities (unwilling or unable carer?)	Should honestly express feelings and needs

Circumstantial factors

Sudden illness

Bed delays

Possible guilt (cause of illness, daughter's lost power to care)

Daughter's exhaustion

Figure 7.3   Frames of reference, nurses and relatives

about routine admissions that prompted the nurse to work with more familiar frames of reference?

By understanding this problem in terms of frames of reference and decision-making as a process, it was then possible to ask how circumstances modified each of these. Decisions necessary in some contexts forced nurses to abandon their working frame of reference. In future projects there was then the possibility that a new frame of reference might be developed for responding to angry relatives. However powerful frames of reference normally were, the group realized why they might have to change suddenly and why this felt stressful for the nurse in such encounters.

Spotting the blind alley

A second important learning issue concerns 'blind alleys'. Blind alleys refer to aspects of your inquiry which have not substantially contributed to the problem solution or practice description. However, this is not to say that journeys down a blind alley have not been fruitful. In many instances, they indicate what is not the case, what should not be considered with reference to similar problems in the future. Spending time examining what prompted your inquiry down a blind alley is therefore important. Which questions and/or evidence prompted you to spend extra time on a part of the analysis? What sustained you in this quest rather longer than it need have done?

Once again, a case example makes the point. A multidisciplinary group of practitioners were working on an EBL study that focused on helping people with learning disabilities to live as independently as possible. The goal of the inquiry was to indicate what the most important dimensions of independence were, and the ways in which different staff understood this concept, contributing help or guidance along the way. The group spent a considerable time debating the notion of holistic care, teasing out in philosophical terms what holism implied and how this influenced the promotion of relative independence among clients with learning disabilities. The group eventually agreed a rather simpler formula for indicating the fit between support measures and client independence (see Figure 7.4).

Initially group work had focused upon different professional conceptions of support or care. Discussions were held about the philosophy of multidisciplinary practice and what the duty of care represented in the context of people with learning disabilities. Upon review, the group decided the turning point was reached when instead of focusing upon philosophy and provision, attention was given to what the client might wish to achieve. This switch had been prompted when the group facilitator suggested that they think of independence as a destination at the end of a car journey. What would this journey take, and how would the various professionals contribute along the way? If the group imagined themselves as a motoring organization, what collective contributions might they offer which would make the journey safe and pleasurable? Figure 7.4 represents this journey. Clients had their own aspirations, some realistic, some less so. Some aspirations were poorly formed or articulated, so that would need work. Independence was partially defined by the client, but relatives also had a say as they dealt with the largest burden of care if the client did not achieve certain self-care abilities. The environmental

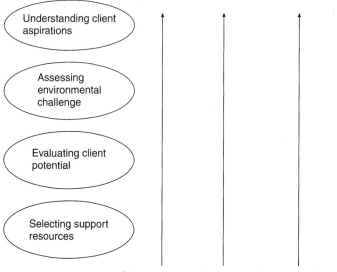

Figure 7.4   Client independence and support

challenge (where the client lived, what support was on offer) set parameters about what might need to be attempted. Environments could be too demanding or undemanding. This prompted the group to discuss motivation and ways of motivating clients. There remained a need to evaluate client potential, learning abilities, preferred ways of learning, ways of dealing with the emotional challenge of change. The combination of these factors was then influenced by available professional resources and the selection of particular ones to suit the client circumstance.

What is informative about this case study is that the group realized that focusing upon the client and an analogy from beyond the boundaries of health care enabled them to break free from arguments that failed to define independence or to suggest how the multidisciplinary team could work together. The motoring analogy was neutral territory to which they could all relate. Presented in simpler terms (as a journey with a destination) helping could be conceived as resourcing, guiding, monitoring and evaluating. What was characteristic of this journey was that the client did not necessarily know how to plan or to evaluate progress. Relatives might need assistance to savour achievement. What was therefore necessary was a support framework flexible enough to suit the client and circumstances.

What had prompted the group down a blind alley were concerns about the completeness of support provision and whether this was philosophically coherent. Coupled to this was the nurses' concern to identify the ways in which other therapist contributions were co-ordinated, so that spiritual, psychological, social as well as physical needs were met. Several therapists failed to understand what could be offered spiritually. There were complex debates about assessing psychological needs, and points made about cognitive ability and emotional readiness to cope with change. It slowly became apparent that the model used to describe work towards independence failed to make sense to all the team members. Efforts meanwhile had been redoubled to make the holistic model explain what they sought collectively to do. It was only when this model was set aside that an alternative way forward could be embraced by all.

Conclusion

Having collected first information and set this down upon the table, it can be daunting to try and analyse it. Even with a group facilitator the process seems difficult and we know that mistakes will be made. The process of analysis is, however, made easier when we remember that the context of our study, its goals and the circumstances under which we look at phenomena help us decide what is relevant or important. Beyond that, we are engaged in evaluating information and deciding whether it can be accepted as fact. Research evidence is associated with evaluative criteria that we may use to judge its merits. Within the confines of these pages it is unrealistic to review all of these, so it is important for investigators to become acquainted with research evaluation as a discipline. This is one of the interfaces between a taught element within a course and the problem-solving group. Beyond this, other claims (information and interpretation) do not come with ready-made evaluative criteria. Before we can accept them as fact, and use them as a basis for further discussion, investigation or conclusions we need to ask searching questions. The process of debating claims and asking such questions is called rhetoric and remains a valuable part of problem- and enquiry-based learning.

Even when we have established what we agree represent facts, however, it is still necessary to reflect upon the ways in which we arrived at these. We need to understand the ways in which we have been investigating and analysing, precisely because this may suggest techniques that we can employ elsewhere. The more aware we are of how we reached conclusions, how we decided what to investigate next, the better able we will be to fashion more artful inquiries in the future. Most health care practice follows this process, although it is rare for practitioners to consider it so consciously. We experience situations, problems, phenomena and try to make sense of them. We have to decide what we think is going on, what can be treated as fact, before we elect to follow a course of action. If we are fortunate, we find opportunity to understand why care measures worked well or seemed to fail. Its now time to consider further investigations within our projects and the ways in which they may reach closure – whether that is a problem solution or an inquiry report.

8 WORKING TOWARDS PROJECT CLOSURE

Having made a series of inquiries, gathered a wealth of information and critically evaluated what has been discovered, the inevitable question arises, 'Where next?' What may have initially seemed a compact problem or a discrete area of practice has tended to 'explode'. We are now aware of many facets of the problem, many dimensions of the practice. If we represented the problem as a spider diagram, with different concepts or issues joined up by arrows indicating influence, our whiteboard image could look extremely tangled. Even when we have decided facts and working theories for what has happened we still ponder how we can manage the analysis so that closure can be reached.

In reality, of course, deciding to close a project, to curtail data gathering and analysis is an artificial cessation of thought. Many health care situations require long-term or incremental analysis, the practitioner returning to the matter periodically. For the purposes of course study, or because colleagues need to move on to other work, there is, however, a need to draw a veil over a project, even if it is recognized that this is a project still left with some loose ends. Listen to three students who talk about working towards closure in problem-based learning contexts:

Ruth: The more you engage in PBL, the more you realize that your problem solution sometimes has to be a best fit one. It's an answer that fits this context and this patient. You wouldn't wish to defend the solution as right in all settings. What enables you to feel good about deciding to stop is that you feel you have a reasonably good grasp of the issues. Your solution fits with the case study you have been looking at.

Sonya: I think of problems as something that expand and contract. They're not static because circumstances change and that means that some aspects of the problem get eroded simply by time. During the analysis of a problem you tend to make the problem bigger, more complex. Then, as you sift through your information again, and check it with a few additional inquiries you start to decide what is important in order to provide a working solution.

Neil: In most of the projects I've been involved in we nudged towards closure, towards deciding what was the best available answer to the question posed. Still, you do reach a point where you feel there is nothing new coming in. You get the problem re-explained in different forms. It's at that point that you think, 'It's time to stop searching now and to summarize what all this means for how I would act.'

We can represent this process using a diagram that not only describes the evolution of projects, but which suggest markers about when it is appropriate to seek closure (see Figure 8.1). Irrespective of whether you are engaged in PBL or EBL study these markers are similar and represent a sea change in what you are attempting to do as a group.

During project mapping your inquiries are directed to finding the edges of the problem or situation, trying to decide just how far the investigation need extend. To use a jigsaw analogy, you are searching for the straight-edged pieces. During the middle part of the project you have begun to examine how some of the information fits together. Some of the images within the jigsaw picture become clear and you search more purposefully for information that is important. Project refinement then represents the effort to fit any last pieces of information together, perhaps

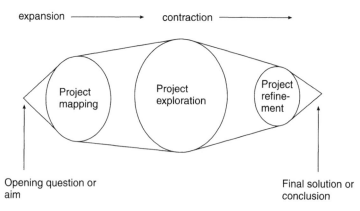

Figure 8.1   The evolution of PBL/EBL projects

answering quite discrete questions. What causes the investigation to expand is new information either being given or discovered and the realization that everyday issues have more dimensions that we expected. We are asking questions for which we do not have instant answers. What causes the investigation to contract is successful analysis where cause and effect are understood or where you appreciate why certain events or experiences happen as they do.

INDICATORS THAT CLOSURE IS NEAR

In Box 8.1 I list some of the indicators that suggest that closure of the investigation may soon be possible. It is assumed for now that you are not simply told that the project has to end and that you have opportunity to wind the project up in a more or less satisfying manner.

Your investigation at this stage has produced a number of tentative solutions or answers, points that will be important

---

Box 8.1   Indicators suggesting closure is near

- There are few new aspects of the problem or practice being discovered through inquiry and/or analysis of the available information.
- You find that you are increasingly able to explain events in terms of cause and effect, what correlates with what and how the environment or context influences what transpires.
- There is increasing consensus about what is desirable, what principles or consideration should guide any final solution or report.
- Any new questions you are posing, any additional information you are gathering is done to verify rather than clarify your ideas. You are offering more confident accounts of why matters have developed in this way and residual questions are there to check out whether your hunch is right.
- You know what sorts of issues or points the final report or problem solution will need to cover.

when all is written up. What you are engaged in now is following last leads in order to verify such statements. The more you are able to confirm that your ideas are accurate and your account reasonably robust, the more refined your final solution or account is likely to be.

VERIFYING WORKING SOLUTIONS OR POINTS

We can illustrate the process of verification with reference to examples in both PBL and EBL.

A PBL example

In the first example the students are working towards a solution concerning how best to assess a client's request for change. The case study refers to a young adult man who has a learning disability and who has started to form a close relationship with a woman (also with learning disability) living within the same communal home. 'Graham' wants to start a sexual relationship with 'Joyce' and staff members are confronted with the problem, how best to respond. In this investigation the study group have ascertained that there are three important components of assessment. These focus upon Graham's and Joyce's capacity to anticipate the possible benefits, responsibilities, problems or need (physical and psychological) that might develop as a result of them having sex together. Fundamentally, the support staff need to ascertain how Joyce feels about Graham's suggestion that they be allowed privacy so that they might make love. This assessment is not solely about intellectual reasoning ability, it also concerns emotional learning. How have Graham and Joyce dealt with strong feelings in the past, how might they respond in the future? Graham has stated that he would take contraceptive precautions. The second aspect of assessment concerns the availability and continuity of support. The communal home represents an environment that might be anticipated to be supportive, but the proposed change may prove stressful for some other residents. During the period of transition, while the relationship between Graham and Joyce either thrives or founders it is likely that key supporters will need to offer additional guidance. Finally, the staff need to understand what Graham and Joyce wish to achieve. If sexual relations are part of a larger and longer-term goal, how can supporters help them to work strategically? If Graham and Joyce are unable to change their environment, for instance, moving to their own accommodation, how can they be assisted to identify goals that are attainable?

In order to verify whether their focus of assessment was correct, the study group decided to run some checks. This involved creating three statements of conditions under which Graham and Joyce might be encouraged to explore their relationship sexually. In the first statement Graham and Joyce were portrayed as cognitively capable of reasoning about the responsibilities of embarking upon a sexual relationship. The couple hoped to form a long-standing relationship and already many of the other residents thought of them as a couple. Unfortunately, however, staff experience in counselling about sexual relationship matters was limited. It was noted that it would be difficult to provide continuity of support from one or two knowledgeable support workers. In the second statement the group adjusted the cognitive capacity variable, indicating that Joyce struggled with concentration and memory and pointing out that she quickly became angry if she felt she was misunderstood by someone she trusted. In the third statement, all three elements were portrayed in favourable light. Study group members then took the statements to expert learning disability practitioners in order to verify what combination of conditions had to be met before a client's request could be supported. They hypothesized that experts would conclude that all three matters had to be favourable before a 'green light' was given. This was confirmed during final interviews, within which the investigators asked experts to 'talk aloud' how they would weigh up their assessment of this situation.

In this verification check the study group was ascertaining whether the planned assessment would seem adequate. They confirmed that all three aspects of assessment (cognitive/emotional ability, a supportive environment and a strategic context) had to be included and criteria met before decisions were made by expert nurses. Remove just one of the components and the decision to support Graham's request was likely to falter. In discussion, the expert nurses observed that cognitive/emotional ability, the potential to learn and grow from a new relationship were the key assessment made. This involved assessing intelligence quotient and emotional readiness.

The group was then ready to propose a solution, which not only stated the foci for assessment in this case study, but which even indicated the relative importance of assessment elements (cognitive/environmental/future goals). The group concluded that decisions in these instances was not solely about ability, but about context and the opportunities the situation afforded to help clients develop their full potential. By assessing what Graham and Joyce hoped to achieve, they could also be involved in decisions that would soon have to be made.

An EBL example

Now let's consider another form of verification, this time concerning the ways in which examiners combine different elements of information in order to mark students' work. This project was being explored by a group of nurse teachers who were concerned about reflective practice and how best to judge what grades to award. They realized that in the end, individual judgement by the tutor was always necessary, but hoped through enquiry-based learning to identify best practice in weighing up the merits of students' work. Figure 8.2 indicates the main factors used by tutors in assessing reflective practice assignments.

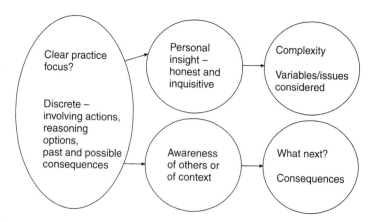

Figure 8.2 Weighing the merits of reflective practice writing

What is significant about this example is the teachers have arranged the components in order. They asked, 'What is most fundamental to evaluating reflection?' The teachers concluded that it was a clear focus upon a practice episode. Without a practice reference point, reflection was just another aspect of philosophy. For reflection to mean something educationally, it had to generate new insights, alternative ideas and then in turn for the student or practice to be changed in some way (Taylor, 2001). Reflection was about the nurses' actions and thought in a context and usually in interplay with others, patients or colleagues, for instance. The study group created a branch of assessment therefore which relied upon clear practice focus but then demonstrated the way in which the nurse explored self, motives, values, premises, and understanding. A competent grade might be awarded for personal insight demonstrated through inquisitive questions about self and motives, choices and decisions. A better mark still might be awarded when this demonstrated the complexity of issues taken into account. These might work in several dimensions: ethical, aesthetic, economic, risk management. The second branch of assessment focused upon contextual awareness. They agreed that teachers awarded marks for work which showed respect for, awareness of others and their interests and needs. Nurses acted in concert with others so it was necessary to think and write in measured and thoughtful terms. Jumping to early or trite conclusions, they agreed, was problematic. What added to marks in this branch of assessment was whether the nurse had anticipated what the episode and his or her actions or inactions might mean for the future.

The group decided to verify their model of assessment by checking a series of previously examined reflective assignments to see whether those students who demonstrated skills in both branches to the end point gained the highest marks. Pairs of teachers read the assignment work independently using the model and then examined the grade awarded by the module tutor. They anticipated that students who started with an incoherent account of the practice would severely damage their chances of a good grade, while those who achieved in one branch of the assessment (either personal insight or contextual awareness) would receive good grades but with some significant discrepancies in marks awarded. The group reached a number of conclusions.

- Writing a clear practice focus was fundamental, students got fail grades when this was done poorly.
- There was wide variance within the grades A–C for students who had demonstrated significant abilities in one or other branch of the assessment.
- No tutor expected students to be equally accomplished in both branches. 'A' grades were awarded for significant achievement in one branch.

This form of verification is not primarily about whether the model is an adequate representation of reality (something done in the PBL example above). Instead, it challenges current practice in order to ascertain whether there is consistency or clarity in assignment marking. The teachers have set a test and found that the model *might* represent best practice but that at this stage the level of reflective writing and grading was not as sophisticated as this. The theory starts to explain why marking reflective work was so difficult and why it was extremely hard to compare marks. While the students weren't being unduly disadvantaged (grades were on the whole fair), neither were they entirely coherent. Teachers would need to debate the relative importance of personal insight and contextual awareness as a feature within reflective writing and the award of grades.

REFINING STATEMENTS

At the end of a project, work focuses not only upon verification but also upon refining of statements. Any account, a solution or explanation of practice must indicate the scholarship of the investigators. Sweeping statements, bold assertions and recommendations bereft of caveats or conditions can mean that the project has been prematurely closed or the group is eager to press a cause that cannot be supported by the available information. In Box 8.2 a number of statements are made at the end of investigations. The investigations were conducted as part of pre-registration courses and indicate varying levels of refinement.

In the first example students were developing an assessment protocol for patients who suffered a loss of consciousness, of unknown origin. The case study dealt with risk management and insofar as it went, study group members had prepared a very

---

Box 8.2   Conclusions (statements) arising out of pre-registration course PBL investigations

1. Intracranial pressure tends to rise following cerebral haemorrhage or trauma. Monitoring for signs of raised intracranial pressure is therefore of critical importance.
2. Clients need a variety of forms of guidance about vaccination against infectious diseases. In some cases vaccination is a requirement (of travel). Advice is therefore 'instructive'. In other cases it is explorative, helping the client make his or her decision in a more informed way. It may also be moral, where guidance supports a course of action protecting the greatest good for the majority, but not necessarily advantageous to the individual.
3. Rapid warming of hypothermic individuals threatens the patient's blood pressure.

---

sound package of assessments and investigations associated with head injuries and pathology such as brain tumours. The study group facilitator though played a role, encouraging students not to foreclose on the possible causes of lost consciousness and reminded them about sub-arachnoid haemmorhage. As statements were prepared, representing a rationale for the neurological assessment package recommended, she challenged the group regarding this statement. She explained that the statement was not entirely comprehensive. It did not accommodate the very different signs and symptoms associated with sub-arachnoid haemorrhage.

Study group facilitators often play a key part, challenging the conclusions that you reach near the end of a project, or the statements that you present in support of a problem solution or practice analysis. Statements may need to be refined either because your group has not brought forward all of the relevant information considered at an earlier stage, or because the choice of statements do not adequately reflect the position that you have adopted. Before projects can be closed, it is necessary to return to your information or even expert sources in order to check points. In this example the problem solution needed to be refined, with additional observations made for the alternative physiological presentation, associated with sub-arachnoid haemorrhage.

The second statement is much more comprehensive and includes recognition that guidance about vaccination is contextual. In some instances members of the public need to be instructed if they are not later to run into difficulties with immigration officials. In other instances the role of the nurse is much more advisory, helping the client to reach his or her well-informed, but personal, decision. This statement is relatively refined. The students who produced this were clear that vaccination advice was by no means 'standard' and that nurses had to understand under what context clients were seeking their help. The statement suggests that these nurses were thinking critically and would be well placed to solve the practice problem – how best to advise travellers about vaccination.

I wonder if you agree with me that 'statement three' needs to be refined a little more, before it becomes part of a problem solution? In this example the students are correct that rapid body warming is dangerous in hypothermia and that this relates to changes in blood pressure. What is not clear, however, is that the group understands why the relationship between body warming and blood pressure is important. The statement requires a short explanation of the underlying rationale. Simply put, rapid warming of the body periphery will cause peripheral vasodilation and a sudden shift of blood to more distant tissues. The core body organs may remain cold in these circumstances and are now adversely affected by a sudden reduction in blood pressure as a result of fluid shift. This can have a profound effect upon heart and respiratory function, threatening the safety of the patient.

In this example the study group solution was to raise body temperature gradually, monitoring core body temperature and explaining the measured intervention to any relatives present. The solution, however, required that the nurses could explain their thinking to onlookers. It is therefore important that statements are refined and underlying rationale available. If you cannot explain your thinking, your solutions might simply be a lucky guess. Just as in mathematics, it is often necessary to show the working out of your equation. Experienced group facilitators are practised in challenging groups about this.

SENSING YOU'VE GOT THERE

Verifying your points, your explanations or solutions, refining your statements is made easier because a group facilitator is available to check your thinking. Within problem- and enquiry-based learning such facilitation is important. If you do not employ, trust or respect the facilitator in such a 'sounding board' role, there is every chance that group members will disagree about what constitutes the final or the best-fit answer. Your group facilitator has this authority either because he or she is trained in the role and appointed by the college, or because you have agreed in advance that the facilitator will act as an arbitrator of final solutions. Provided that he or she has listened attentively and allowed you to develop your own exploration (rather than tell you what to think or decide), the group facilitator will be well placed to confirm that your investigation has reached a reasonable coda.

Beyond such independent evaluation, however, students often attest to personal feelings and thoughts that help confirm that learning has taken place. This is often referred to in terms of levels of understanding or an appreciation of just why the health care world seems as it is. Here are some quotes that typify that 'ah hah' moment:

> *Susan*: I knew we'd got it when I was on the ward and rehearsing our explanation of stigma to a psychologist there. I was able to give examples of why it occurred, how it felt and what function it served for others, if not the poor old sufferer. The psychologist was impressed and said, OK, then, tell me about Mrs X in terms of stigma – what's going on in her situation then? I could answer. I could explain a lot of Mrs X's problem in terms of stigma. She didn't just have an illness, she had a label. The psychologists congratulated me and I got this real glow about what I knew.

> *Janice*: What I like is when your project reaches the end and you can explain just why something is the way it is. That's not to say that you're arrogant about it, it's just that you know why things are not straightforward. One of our projects was about rehabilitating stroke victims. I understood what potential the nervous system has to compensate for damage, how therapists help patients learn after a stroke and what the limitations of a rehabilitation service are. They add up in varying measures to what state the patient is in 12 months after a CVA.

In Susan's case she has received external verification of her understanding. Not only has she understood the concept of stigma but she also knows how to use it as a tool to understand different patient's circumstances. She senses the freedom that this provides, because the concept might apply in many different settings (e.g. sexually transmitted disease, mental illness). As you reach the final stages of your group investigation it is common to rehearse your thinking aloud with others and in many projects you will hear again and again what a succinct and incisive grasp of the situation you appear to have. Getting these sorts of messages can help to reinforce your confidence and confirm that the investigation has not lost its way.

In Janice's case the sense of arrival is perhaps more personal. She has looked at the rehabilitation 'track records' of different patients and confronted her own feelings and confusion concerning why some patients seemed to progress better than others. Altruistically Janice hoped to see every patient attain a high degree of independence. Realistically, however, people suffered different sorts of cerebrovascular accidents in different parts of the brain and with varying capacity to recover. Rehabilitation support and training were part of the equation but not the only one. Understanding what was involved in rehabilitation and what determined the progress of individual patients enabled her to make a more objective evaluation of nursing care. Fundamentally, by understanding the factors influencing patient progress she felt better able to cope with working in an environment where not every outcome was a perfect one.

CONCLUSION

Reaching closure in a project involves arriving at explanations of what is going on (EBL) or solutions to problems (PBL) which seem coherent to facilitators and other verifiers. Closure involves a sense of personal satisfaction, of feeling that you have learned something significant, which may be of practical use in other contexts in the future. As the project contracts and you select only those explanations, which seem right or best fit for the situation, it becomes important to try out your account of what has been observed or discovered. This chapter has provided examples of how you might verify your answers, but these are not exhaustive. Your group facilitator may well suggest other ways in which you can verify whether your account is reasonable, whether your solution seems appropriate for the problem in hand.

Whatever your final explanation, however, it is usually necessary to refine the statements which go to make it up. This may involve demonstrating that your account is measured, adding explanations of why the situation is as it is or demonstrating that you understand processes underway. Simply put, projects lead to statements that explain what is happening and why. In the case of problem-based learning this extends to solutions, suggestions concerning what might be done to resolve the difficulty or to ameliorate the situation. In these terms, what you have produced (with due guidance and help) are statements that go beyond intuition. You articulate what has been observed, why you would behave as you do and under what conditions you might adjust your explanation or solution. These are very significant achievements within health care work!

So far so good. It is now to time to consider just what forms assessment might take and how you might defend your conclusions. If you have been conducting your project as part of a programme of study, module assessments come along soon enough. If you have been investigating outside the college context, there are still others that you may need to convince of your findings.

9 PREPARING FOR ASSESSMENT

For the purposes of this chapter, the term assessment will be used in its widest sense, referring to any form of external judgement on the adequacy (or otherwise) of learning or progress, associated with problem- or enquiry-based projects. Assessments take different formats and can include coursework and examinations (educational programme-related learning) as well as reports (frequently an end product in non-course related EBL). In educational programmes assessment is often of the individual nurse, precisely because it is difficult to assess contributions within group work. Marks-Maran and Thomas (2000) summarize many of the assessment and evaluation methods associated with problem-based learning and some of these have been adopted or adapted for use within EBL. In some instances familiar and standard forms of assessment are attached to problem- and enquiry-based learning curricula. This is usually less satisfactory as such assessments emphasize assessment of accrued knowledge rather than skill development. What the more authentic PBL/EBL assessment methods tend to share are the following:

- An evaluation of content knowledge, your command of information and empirical data.
- Assessment of your investigative processes, the ways in which you analyse a problem or explore a practice issue.
- Exploration of your ability to adapt your thinking to the prevailing circumstances. Many problems (and their solutions) are contextual so it is important to couch assessments in terms of case studies and developing situations.

In this chapter we will take each of the assessment formats in turn, describe what is characteristic about it and suggest practical ways in which you can respond to the challenges set by your examiners. In hybrid forms of assessments, devised by particular university departments, it may be necessary to adapt your approach and here I recommend consultation with your tutor.

THE MODIFIED ESSAY QUESTION (MEQ)

Modified essay questions were first devised within medical education and designed to assess not only the practitioners' factual knowledge but the process of assessment, diagnosis and planning intervention (Hodgkin and Knox, 1975). Knox (1980) explains that modified essays should explore the attitudes as well as the knowledge of practitioners. This is important within health care professions, where the approach to situations and clients may be as important as knowledge employed. In basic form the modified essay question begins with a case study that describes a situation. In the case of problem-based learning this includes one or more pieces of information which suggests that all is not well, or that there is potential for some form of tension, perhaps a deterioration in the patient's circumstances, or conflict between the interests of different stakeholders. In most PBL curricula the case study is based on a patient story, although there are no reasons why the case study cannot be a staff problem involving the interests of colleagues rather than clients. In the case of enquiry-based learning curricula the introductory scenario may not focus upon a particular patient, client or colleague, but upon a practice field or area. Here the opening scenario suggests that practice is missing some form of knowledge or skill and you are invited to explore what might underpin, enrich or enhance practice.

What is typical of the MEQ is that you are invited to write down your opening response to the scenario presented. This usually takes the form of a summary of what you understand the situation to be about, what seems problematic or unclear and what measures might be necessary to press forward your investigation of the circumstances prevailing. It's really rather like an opening chess move. Your examiner wants to understand whether you think strategically and can move in ways that enable you to operate most effectively, especially as matters become clearer. He or she is not trying to catch you out, however, because incrementally new snippets of information are added. You are invited to respond with new ideas and information, suggesting not only what you understand is important, but how you will use information in order to deal with the developing situation (Silen, 1998). To ensure that the assessment is fair, a panel of subject and practice skill experts is asked to critically read the case study and the series of developing information and questions. The panel identifies what constitute reasonable responses. The essays are carefully devised to assess the scope of your knowledge, your ability to organize yourself answering each part of the case study in turn and to evaluate your concept analysis or problem-solving skills.

Figure 9.1 summarizes a modified question essay that might be used as part of a nurse education curriculum. In Figure 9.1 notice how the patient story line is set out in stages, together with the sorts of practice skills that will be assessed *en route*.

Marsha's story	
Admitted via casualty from a 'squat', Marsha is confused and shows signs of bruising on her arms. She is malnourished.	Opening scenario designed to assess your ability to evaluate the situation and the range and seriousness of problems that Marsha might face. It also challenges you to demonstrate your attitude towards this patient and the establishment of a patient–nurse relationship.
Marsha has been in a fight and was knocked unconscious. She is admitted for observations.	You're now given more information which focuses in upon a particular trauma problem. You must demonstrate your understanding of head injuries, neurological observations while keeping in mind other variables that could affect your observations.
Marsha's neurological condition deteriorates rapidly. She shows signs of raised intracranial pressure. What next!	The case study now tests your ability to act decisively, requesting assistance as appropriate and managing risk. You must demonstrate your appreciation of altered physiology and why the signs of raised intracranial pressure are so critical. You must stabilize the situation working with other colleagues to assist Marsha.

Figure 9.1   Modified essay question

In the case of enquiry-based learning curricula MEQs have a similar evolutionary character, with incremental information added for you to examine and respond to. For example, you may first be advised that colleagues have expressed an interest in developing a set of ethical guidelines for advising mothers about immunization. While there is already a literature on the risks associated with childhood infections and a growing array of reports on the safety of vaccinations, there seems rather less material on the ethics of health promotion in this context. In stage one of this MEQ you are then challenged to 'scope' what aspects of ethical practice your investigation might need to cover. You are asked to indicate what principles or frameworks might need to be taken into account. In stage two of this MEQ you are advised that the group has begun to focus upon 'informed consent'. You are now challenged to debate what constitutes informed consent and to consider the various attitudes or world-views among staff that might influence how this issue is approached. In stage 3 of the MEQ you are given a 10-point ethics guideline relating to this issue and asked to discuss how you would verify whether the guideline was coherent and workable.

Tackling the MEQ depends in part upon whether you have all the elements of information available at the outset, or whether these are issued at various stages within the assessment. In examinations, for instance, you may be allocated a set number of minutes to each section of your analysis, before another piece of information is provided to you. In coursework assessment, you may receive your developing case study piecemeal. It is then clearly important to work on the first sections of the study, making best use of the available time. However tempting it might be to wait until the whole scenario unfolds before writing, you should make a start, answering the first questions when they arrive. Your examiners appreciate that some of what you offer within the first section will not be developed in later sections. For instance, in the example of Marsha above (Figure 9.1), you might write initially about assessing her nutritional state, whether she has a drugs-related problem and whether living in squat conditions means that she is suffering from an infestation. In later sections only the drug abuse angle might be revisited, precisely because use of drugs might affect Marsha's neurological status.

A well-constructed MEQ mimics in large degree the investigative journey that you have been making in previous projects during your course. To answer them effectively it is worth recalling the range of issues, and the investigative skills that were important in such projects. The fact that you may not have encountered a 'Marsha' in your past group work should not unduly panic you. Provided that you have gleaned information about neurological assessment, living conditions and principles of health assessment and patient history taking in other contexts, it should be possible to bring relevant ideas to bear in this setting. In tackling MEQs it is then useful to remember three principles when preparing your answers:

1. Do not jump to conclusions. While opening information remains vague, consider all the possible interpretations of the situation that seem possible. Try not to label the patient or pre-empt other possible explanations for what has been happening.
2. Remember that nursing care is also about attitude and approach. Try to convey sensitivity within your answer – a concern for other stakeholders in the situation. In most MEQ patient scenarios, the patient is in a vulnerable position.
3. Acknowledge the expertize of others and the limitations of your role or situation. Consider whether a referral or second opinion might assist you in this scenario. Please note, however, that adding a remark such as, 'I would ask the doctor's opinion on this' to each and every question is likely to attract censure to your work. Nursing involves risk assessment and an appreciation of what you yourself can offer.

THE TRIPLE JUMP TEST

The triple jump test is most commonly associated with problem-based learning and is usually conducted as a modified form of viva (Painvin *et al.*, 1979; Pallie and Carr, 1987). Your own tutor, or another academic colleague, presents you with a case scenario, which involves one or more problems. You are invited to make an initial assessment of the situation and to suggest what you think may be some of the most critical issues involved. Your examining tutor will use a series of probing questions designed to help you 'tease out' what is important within the situation. The whole of this process then represents step 1 within the triple jump. In step 2 you are given time and resources with which to explore the situation further. The purpose of step 2 is to provide you with further 'fuel' for your analysis and quite frequently to develop an account of how you would act in this situation. You are usually free to make notes and to highlight which bits of information you will rely upon to support your arguments for what you would do next. In step 3 of the triple jump you return to the viva in order to present your revised or updated analysis of the situation and your account of how and why you would proceed in a particular way. In this part of the viva you will need to defend your thinking, and explain how you are using critical pieces of information in order to explain your approach. To ensure that all students are assessed equitably, the step 1 probe questions used by your assessor are usually pre-set and designed to help all students demonstrate their analysis to the full. All students receive the same resources in step 2 and a set of criteria are developed by a panel of experts to indicate what will be considered successful answers in step 3. Because your answers are usually verbal, it is then important that a second assessor is present to verify how your answers are interpreted and graded.

In Figure 9.2 you will see a summary of one triple jump assessment taken from a problem-based learning context. The assessment in this instance lasted 120 minutes, with 30 minutes allocated to the step 1 opening assessment of a scenario, 60 minutes allocated to the review of resource material and planning a revised/updated response and 30 minutes allocated to presentation of your plan of action. Like all vivas it can be potentially stressful, although tutors work hard to put you at your ease and to help you present your thinking in best possible light. Preparing for such a viva revolves around three activities.

Revising relevant syllabus knowledge

This form of assessment is necessarily focused on one scenario, one part of the syllabus. Nevertheless, it usually exists within a module of study or you may be forewarned of the field of practice that the scenario is concerned with. Your assessors are not hoping to test your encyclopaedic knowledge on all

Scenario	Probe questions
An elderly patient is admitted to the burns unit with 30 per cent burns after falling asleep while smoking a cigarette in bed. As he arrives on your ward his airway is secure and an intravenous infusion has been started. The gentleman has been catheterized. The burns have been suffered on both arms, the upper chest and to one side of his face.	Why is this patient 'at risk?' In what ways does the fact that he is a cigarette smoker possibly complicate his condition? What homeostatic principles are being addressed through the use of intra-venous fluids and the use of a urinary catheter? How does pain figure your assessment?

Resources	Instructions
Burns charts and guidelines on assessing fluid replacement regime Papers on pain and analgesia in acute burns settings A short guide to burns dressings in different parts of the body.	Prepare your plan of action regarding this patient for the next four hours of your shift. Indicate how you will prioritize your work.

Student presentation	Probe questions
Sustaining airway Managing homeostatic balance Dealing with pain Providing psychological support Monitoring Dressing wounds (if not already achieved)	Summarize what you would do during this period. What physiological concerns are you dealing with through these measures? What psychological issues are you dealing with here? What evidence is there to support your choice of action?

Figure 9.2   Summary of a triple jump test

things nursing. They want to know whether you can use relevant information to practical effect. With this in mind, it is worth revising your knowledge of relevant subject matter, for instance, problems of pregnancy, cancer chemotherapy, dealing with depression, whatever is the focus of the module.

Rehearsing reasoning

A viva is a performance within which you rehearse aloud your reasoning. As with any other performance there is advantage in conducting rehearsals. In this instance this is achieved by working with one or more colleagues and creating case studies, scenarios of your own. A friend acts as the question master and probes your understanding of the situation described. You are then free to consult one or more colleagues (your resource) before returning to your inquisitor in order to present your plan of action. The process of creating a scenario of your own is itself instructive. You learn about what could be problematic within any setting. Your colleagues learn from the answers that you provide. In these terms the study group benefits from collective rehearsal sessions.

Practising your critical reading

Within the triple jump test you will normally be provided with some reading to complete. There will be only a limited time within which to conduct this, extracting the most important points that you can then use within your plan or defence of approach. For this reason it is useful to select example articles, policies or other papers on subjects within your module and to then practise identifying the five most important facts from each. Highlight the facts that seem most important, ask a colleague to read the paper and then defend to her or him how you would employ this information within a defence of care associated.

PORTFOLIOS OF LEARNING

Both of the above forms of assessment suffer a key limitation. They focus their attention upon a very discrete part of the syllabus and do not provide opportunities for examiners to test your coverage of other relevant subject matter. For this reason, such assessments are often combined with conventional examinations and/or multiple choice question tests which attend to subject knowledge. They may also be combined, as part of coursework, with the challenge to produce a portfolio of your learning. Portfolios of learning vary in their design and format and are influenced by the university's assessment aims. In general, however, portfolios usually include at least three elements:

- Descriptions of practice experience, episodes of care or themes relating to practice.
- Written account of your reflections upon such matters. This usually includes a first impressions account of the situation or subject and subsequent and more refined assessments of the situation.
- Either action plans and or descriptions of your nursing care response. Care delivery is then regularly evaluated to ascertain whether the problem is being addressed/resolved or whether the practice is now better understood.

In portfolios of learning you decide which episodes or aspects of practice to include, which case studies of care you will follow through. The university may require you to submit your whole portfolio or only what you consider the best of your work associated with a module. Portfolios may be summatively assessed (that is for the award of marks and grades) at the end of each module, or at the end of each year (when module assessments of the portfolio are considered formative). Typically you are invited to work upon your portfolio with a designated personal tutor or mentor, someone who will take an interest in the development of your professional skills and command of subject matter.

In Figure 9.3 several different forms of portfolio are highlighted. These may be used in problem- or enquiry-based learning. In some university settings marking is completed by a tutor, while in others there is some element of self- or peer group assessment. In the latter case a percentage of the available marks (say, 10–20 per cent) are awarded by your peers who are encouraged to develop their constructive and critical faculties by examining your coursework. To ensure that marking is equitable, clear marking guidelines are set and cross-marking is avoided (limiting the chance that colleagues will simply swap good marks one for another). If you are invited to self-assess your own work, a tutor will normally be allocated to help you reach as objective an evaluation as possible.

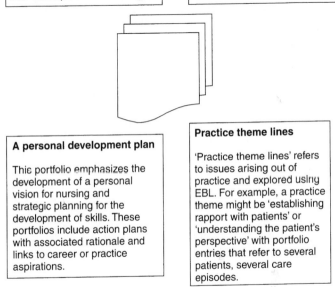

Based on care episodes

Often these are grounded in one or other model of reflection and completed in association with a clinical supervisor. The goal is to help you demonstrate the building of theory from practice and the subsequent adjustment of practice in the light of your new-found practice knowledge.

Based upon transferable skills

The university identifies key transferable skills which must be demonstrated in your exploration of care episodes or practice issues. For example, effective information retrieval using databases and human sources of information.

A personal development plan

This portfolio emphasizes the development of a personal vision for nursing and strategic planning for the development of skills. These portfolios include action plans with associated rationale and links to career or practice aspirations.

Practice theme lines

'Practice theme lines' refers to issues arising out of practice and explored using EBL. For example, a practice theme might be 'establishing rapport with patients' or 'understanding the patient's perspective' with portfolio entries that refer to several patients, several care episodes.

Figure 9.3   Types of portfolio

In planning your own portfolio entries it is important to clarify just which form of portfolio is being requested by the university. Check any instructions very carefully and ask relevant questions of your personal tutor or clinical supervisor before you commit lots of entries to your folder. Once you have done this, select care episodes that seem to exemplify important or interesting aspects of nursing practice. Recording everything you see or do is impractical, so before you write, pause and answer the question, 'Why would my entry be useful to myself, or another practitioner, several months hence?' Episodes of care or aspects of practice that are usually worthy of reflection include the following:

- Those that have proven very successful in terms of care process or client outcome (why did this work so well?).
- Those that have forced you to re-examine your previous perceptions or attitudes (does what I do, or how I think make sense in this context too?).
- Those which exemplify how a particular context or new intervening factors cause health care professionals to adjust their strategies (for example, how does the patient's ethnic culture influence patient education? How does care within the patient's own home modify the risk assessment made by a nurse?).
- Those which you believe have assisted you to practise in more imaginative or sensitive ways.
- Those which exemplify where research evidence has purchase upon practice.
- Those that cause you to re-evaluate your education, the theory or philosophy that you have previously been taught.

In Figure 9.4 a flow chart is used to describe the way in which one nurse developed her own portfolio. In this instance she was free to design her own work, provided that it demonstrated a critical attitude towards her own practice and offered opportunities for examiners to appreciate how she had used a variety of resources to think afresh about her nursing approach. In this example, Elaine *could* have simply accumulated a series of reflective practice episodes that were only loosely related insofar as they occurred in the same clinical placement. More imaginatively, however, Elaine develops two threads of inquiry within her portfolio that has many of the characteristics of inquisitive, enquiry-based learning.

In making portfolio entries it is important to write enough detail about the practice episode to enable your reader to understand the context within which events happened. In the following example, description B is rather better than A, even though both accounts are relatively succinct. This is because description B incorporates more details about what the nurse herself was doing. Understanding roles is usually important if care episodes are to be adequately evaluated. Notice too how

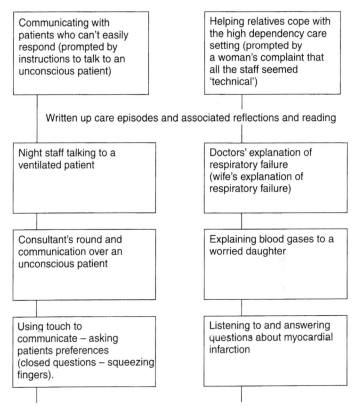

Communicating with patients who can't easily respond (prompted by instructions to talk to an unconscious patient)	Helping relatives cope with the high dependency care setting (prompted by a woman's complaint that all the staff seemed 'technical')

Written up care episodes and associated reflections and reading

Night staff talking to a ventilated patient	Doctors' explanation of respiratory failure (wife's explanation of respiratory failure)
Consultant's round and communication over an unconscious patient	Explaining blood gases to a worried daughter
Using touch to communicate – asking patients preferences (closed questions – squeezing fingers).	Listening to and answering questions about myocardial infarction

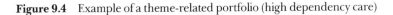

Self-initiated essay – 'Levels and styles of communication, understanding those who can't or don't speak the same language'.

Figure 9.4 Example of a theme-related portfolio (high dependency care)

description B offers a simple explanation of thought as well as action. In the description this is neither defended nor damned. It is presented as a simple description of omission:

Description A

'Ursula' was admitted to the ward just before shift handover. The night staff was coming on duty. Ursula was clearly distressed, crying and saying how stupid she had felt taking the overdose of analgesics. She complained of discomfort, resulting from the tube that had been used to 'wash the tablets out of her stomach'. She wondered where her daughters were and what they might think of her actions. However much she hated their father, she felt she was proving a wretched mother, behaving as she had. A staff nurse colleague and I helped Ursula into bed and then washed her face and hands, assisting her to feel fresher. My colleague stepped outside of the bay to answer a bleep and was overheard confiding to another nurse what a nuisance 'such admissions were at a shift handover'. I immediately dismissed this complaint to Ursula, who had overheard the comment and was now close to tears once more.

Description B

The incident associated with 'Ben' happened soon after 4 a.m., when I was checking patients on the ward, as one of two night staff available. My colleague was a care assistant who did regular nights. Ben had been admitted after a cerebrovascular accident and during the previous days had been making a slow but steady recovery. To date he had slept well at night. On this occasion, however, he awoke agitated calling for his wife. I went quickly to him, trying to reassure him that 'Margaret' would see him in the morning. I pulled the cot sides of the bed up and asked my colleague to check the remaining patients. As I pulled up the cot sides my first concern was for Ben's safety. I elected to remain by his bedside until he had settled. What I had not done was to consider how the darkness and Ben's stroke had served to disorientate him. I did not try to reorientate him to where he was, who I was and why he was now safe.

Following this, you need to present an account of reasoning behind the action or inaction. If your studies have been conducted in terms of problem-based learning it is necessary to explain what was problematic about the care episode. What tensions existed between the two nurses in description A above and why care was perhaps more superficial in description B. In the following excerpt from description B notice how this nurse considers a number of dimensions regarding what she had and had not done with regard to 'Ben'.

Description B (continued)

Standing beside Ben's bed and watching him slowly subside back into sleep I pondered what could have made that care better. Some of my answers came to me later, but they all started with trying to imagine what that night awakening must have seemed like for Ben. It was dark, but there was some noise at the far end of the ward. A monitor bleeped, there were whispered voices. Whose were they? Where am I? I needed to think about:

1. What had prompted Ben's awakening? What happens in the mind as the brain slowly compensates for a stroke?
2. Did the awakening and disorientation signify progress of some sort?
3. What was the most important information to give Ben, enough to reassure him without waking other patients?
4. Would touch have reassured him? Ben didn't know me especially well, as this was my second night on and he'd not been awake the previous night.

In this student's case the questions prompted an interview with a psychologist and reading about sleep–wake patterns among patients recovering from neurological problems. These were written up as resource evidence before she once again returned to her portfolio, writing an account of how she would now approach a disorientated patient at night. The list included, speaking in a soft voice, saying who you were first of all. It included reminding the patient where he was and that this was a safe place. Touch the patient's arm (a socially acceptable place to use touch) and then hold the hand firmly. Provide answers to his questions, reassuring him about what will happen next or soon. Disorientation has several different dimensions, time, place, the sequence and significance of recent events and those about to happen next.

PREPARING A REPORT

Some form of written report is the most usually assessed outcome of an enquiry-based learning project conducted outside an educational course. Price, A. (2000a, b, 2001a, b) provides useful summaries of the different forms that a report could take. These include evaluative, feasibility and process report forms. While these articles refer to consultancy, it is not unreasonable to draw upon them for EBL contexts, when we consider that a line manager may be the recipient of the study group's findings following an investigation. Evaluative reports provide a critical review of a service, state of practice development or care delivery. They explain the context of the enquiry and then elucidate just what is being provided and what progress has been made over time. Feasibility reports are written when either the group or the manager is considering new ways of conducting care, delivering a service. They report upon what issues need to be considered before a plan can be actioned. Process reports are rather 'softer' in style and report on the evolution of ideas, approaches, frames of reference used by a group with regard to a particular subject or practice. They provide the reader with an insight into the 'care culture', the ways in which group members think about what they do.

What the reader needs to understand from your report is the following:

- What prompted the enquiry, why was it important to do (sometimes this is called the terms of reference).
- What the group set out to investigate and over what time frame.
- What information sources were used, which stakeholders or experts were consulted.
- How the investigation progressed, what were your lines of inquiry?
- What conclusions have been reached.
- What future action is recommended (this may include further investigations or it might suggest changes in practice where there is strong collective support for the same).

To help the reader find her or his way quickly around your document, I suggest that you adopt a crisp and business-like style that distils many of the debates, arguments and dead ends that a typical enquiry may have gone through. You will achieve this if you adopt the following approach to your writing:

- Use a clear title that sums up your investigation.
- Provide an abstract/executive summary of the investigation at the start (3–4 paragraphs should be enough).
- Create an index and number your pages.
- Don't overburden the work with references (include summary of references and source evidence within appendices so that this does not detract from the narrative).
- Use tables and diagrams to get points across quickly (e.g. a flow chart to explain the sequence of your investigation).

- Number your sections and the subsections that follow within it. For instance, 2.3.2 refers to subsection 2, of section 3, within part 2 of a report. You can then use these numbers when making a cross-reference for the reader to refer to.
- Make sure that your conclusions and recommendations stem out of the body of information, and associated evidence that you present within your report. Conclusions and recommendations should not extend beyond what you have explained in previous sections, nor should they 'arrive out of the blue'.
- Explain the group's progress, the group's conclusions. Do not confuse matters by referring to what each member thought or suggested.
- Check with colleagues whether the work seems an authentic representation of the investigation and the conclusions before you offer it to anyone else for perusal.
- Make sure you have permission to include any relevant statistics, illustrations or tables from stakeholders, especially experts that you may have consulted.

It is unrealistic to reproduce a whole report within a chapter of this length. Such reports may extend to between 5000 and 10,000 words depending on the nature and the length of an investigation. In any case no sample report can adequately illustrate all report situations. In Figure 9.5 therefore you will see the outline of a report, by section, which refers to the management of abusive patients or relatives within a group practice setting. The outline provides a useful impression of what sorts of information was included and the length of the work involved.

It may surprise you to discover just how much your group discussions can be distilled, when it is accepted that you present only that which is left after the debates. Students who have completed such reports typically suggest that the report seems to represent some 20 per cent of the effort that went into the investigation. Much of what you have considered and discarded remains hidden. The one exception to this observation occurs within process reports, where the account includes an explanation of the evolution of ideas. Here, flow charts are often employed to suggest how thinking has become more focused, more refined. This said, a process report does not warrant sloppy writing. The reader needs to understand the journey you

Summary (rationale for investigation)	3
Contents page and list of resources accessed	4
1. Investigation process	6
1.1 Description of methods employed	8
1.2 Stakeholders accessed	11
1.3 Expertize accessed	12
1.4 Use of databases	13
2. Key terms employed	15
3. Complaints and abusive episodes	16
3.1 Incidence of verbal abuse (2002)	17
3.2 Incidence of physical violence (2002)	18
3.3 Contexts of violence (2002)	18
4. Reading angry people, volatile situations	20
4.1 Preceding influences	20
4.2 Environmental influences	21
4.3 Professional-triggered influences	23
5. Forestalling violence	24
5.1 Giving attention	24
5.2 Asking questions/making judgements	26
5.3 Giving advice	27
5.4 Emergency measures	29
6. Conclusion	31
7. Recommendations	33
Appendix 1 (Statistics on assault/violent behaviour 1999–2001)	35
Appendix 2 (Hospital protocol – handling aggression)	37
Appendix 3 (Selected and annotated research evidence papers)	39

Figure 9.5 Example of an evaluative report format

made without undue pause to debate discrete points at every juncture.

Conclusion

While assessment of any form of learning can be a daunting prospect, that associated with problem- and enquiry-based learning usually mimics the process of learning that has been employed *en route*. Modified essay questions and triple jump tests replicate the stages of thinking and inquiry typically employed within the study group. Portfolios represent a similar concern, focusing upon reflection and inductive learning. While they are completed as an individual, they include the possibility of consultation with a clinical supervisor, personal tutor or mentor. Reports provide the group with a chance, through a secretary or report author, to represent what has been learned.

Assessment is necessary within academic programmes to evaluate student progress and, by implication, the success or otherwise of teaching and group facilitation. It represents an artificial hiatus because in practice problem-solving is a cyclical progress, during which nurses repeatedly modify their stance, the care they give to patients. Nevertheless, assessment affords study group members an opportunity for feedback. Beyond the grade or percentage mark, there are often valuable reflections and observations upon the process by which you arrived at your conclusions and action plans. In many regards this is the most valuable and long-term reward for submitting yourself to assessment. Good quality feedback might prompt adjustments to your practice.

Success in assessment is founded first in completing problem- and enquiry-based learning in an engaged way. The more you immerse yourself in the process, the better equipped you will be to answer EBL or PBL questions. Beyond that, however, rehearsing the process of enquiry or problem-solving is also valuable. Not only should this help you to manage your nerves before assessment but it might also help colleagues to revise vicariously for their assessments too.

Part III

TWO CASE STUDIES

In this part of the textbook I present two case studies, one drawn from problem-based learning and one drawn from enquiry-based learning. The purpose of such case studies is not to instruct you how inquiry *should* take place. Rather, they are included to illustrate the challenges faced by study groups, the ups and downs of inquiry and the ways in which projects were developed. Necessarily the case studies exist within a particular field of practice. Your own may differ from these, but what I hope you will nonetheless gain from reading them is a richer understanding of inquiry process. They represent successful case studies to the extent that they help you overcome your anxieties and appreciate why problem- or enquiry-based learning represents a challenging but also rewarding way to learn.

10 A PROBLEM-BASED LEARNING CASE STUDY

This case study was devised using the experiences of a number of patients rehabilitating after suffering facial burns. The condition of patients at this stage has been stabilized. Their physical health has been much improved through the ministrations of staff on the burns unit. Ahead of them, however, lies the psychological challenges of returning to the outside world – family, friends, the environment beyond the burns and plastic surgery unit that may have come to represent a protective cocoon (see Pruzinsky, 1998, for further information). In this case study post-registration nurses explored the rehabilitation journey with particular emphasis upon psycho-social care associated with disfigurement. The case study was presented because it highlighted the challenges associated with rehabilitation in a number of different circumstances where physical appearance is rapidly and often radically altered.

PAUL'S STORY

The study group was presented with the story of Paul, a young soldier who had suffered burns to his face and upper torso after rescuing a colleague from a burning patrol vehicle. In Box 10.1 the opening scenario and associated questions are presented.

Box 10.1   Opening scenario

Forgive me if my writing seems a bit scrawled – my right hand got burned in the fire, just like my face, the side of my neck and the front of my chest. I dragged John, my mate, clear and we both got left with burns. The Commanding Officer called me a hero and

---

Box 10.1   (continued)

back in the burns unit, when they were patching me up, I believed him. I think that idea kept me going, that I'd got these injuries because I was doing something right for once. I've been in the army now for just over three years. I've done time in Northern Ireland and further afield, even seen a fair bit of action, but none of that prepared me for this. While I was in the burns unit the pain was incredible. They did their best, but the burns hurt like hell, and when I finally looked in the mirror I had a face liked a melted wax crayon.

My fiancée is called Siobhan. She'd been with me for nearly a year and visited me most days while I really ill. She used to scold me when I complained about my treatment. 'Don't be such a kid', she would say. I could tell her anger was a way of coping. If she told me off, it gave her a role, something important to work at. 'Take each day at a time', she told me. Funny though, I don't think she was doing that herself. She must have always been wondering what we would do when all the intensive care was over. What would we do when it was time for me to go home and convalesce for a while?

Questions

1. What is your assessment of Paul's psychological state now as he begins a period of rehabilitation beyond the burns unit, but still on the 'burns and plastics' ward?
2. What are the risks that Paul will suffer an 'altered body image'?
3. How might you assess Paul's available support during the forthcoming weeks?

PRELIMINARY APPRAISAL

The study group's preliminary appraisal of this situation focused upon three issues. The first was what experience they had of disfigurement and rehabilitation, in any setting, whether related to burns or elsewhere. One group member had worked on an oncology ward where surgery had sometimes been radical, while a second nurse had worked in casualty where she had witnessed initial reactions to injuries by relatives. Beyond that, they had relatively little experience of this situation. The second issue concerned what they currently understood about psychological states, including 'altered body image' (see Price, 1995, for a further appraisal). Once again, two study group members knew a little about reactive depression, although they claimed no special knowledge of altered body image. The third issue identified was concerned with making assessments of a patient's psychological state and level of support. They agreed that their previous experience had been in assessing the physical status of patients and/or their living conditions. The group therefore reluctantly concluded that any 'first impressions' of this problem would be commonsensical rather than professionally informed. They would need to consult some experts and complete some further reading very quickly indeed.

The group began by trying to imagine how it would feel to deal with a facial burn, after the life-threatening stage of the injury was over. They used a flipchart in order to map these preliminary ideas out (see Figure 10 1).

The group then reviewed what they considered to be the facts of the case. Paul had a fiancée who to date had seemed very supportive. They nonetheless decided that facial burns were potentially very damaging for morale. Individuals associated themselves with facial appearance as was illustrated by the fact that most portraiture was 'head and shoulders' focused. They considered it a fact that cosmetic surgery could improve physical function and improve appearance. This said, they thought it naïve to imagine that all signs of facial scarring could be obliterated. Paul would live with a new, and possibly a less attractive face for the rest of his life.

There were a number of learning issues apparent within the problem described. The first of these was to understand the level of psychological risk associated with facial burns (Franklin *et al.*, 1996, provide a review of cosmetic outcomes). At the extreme the group decided that patients might become suicidal. At the very least, the patient would have to think afresh about how he managed social encounters with others. The second issue was associated with altered body image. What did this concept involve? How did you recognize altered body image within a patient? It struck the group that the third learning issue was best investigated

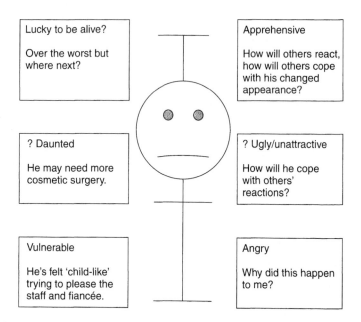

Lucky to be alive?

Over the worst but where next?

Apprehensive

How will others react, how will others cope with his changed appearance?

? Daunted

He may need more cosmetic surgery.

? Ugly/unattractive

How will he cope with others' reactions?

Vulnerable

He's felt 'child-like' trying to please the staff and fiancée.

Angry

Why did this happen to me?

Figure 10.1   A rough impression of Paul's psychological state

last. The level of support that a patient might hope for seemed to depend in part upon understanding the psychological damage inflicted (see also, Kleve and Robinson, 1999). Angry patients for instance might be hard to love. Angry or depressed patients might also find it hard to accept help from others, particularly if this was misconstrued as charity.

The group agreed four lines of inquiry. These were agreed on the basis that the experience of burns was a personal and changing one. For that reason it was important to ask those who had witnessed such change about the stress and coping. Equally, however, there was a need to understand abstract concepts, such as altered body image and support.

1. How does psychological state change after acute stage of burns? How do you assess this? (Sources of expertise: burns and plastics ward staff, especially those with outpatient experience. Articles within specialist journals, including *Rehabilitation Nursing*, suggested as possible sources of illustration by the group facilitator.)

2. What is altered body image? (Sources of expertize: subject search within the library. Review of web sites dealing with 'disfigurement'.)
3. What is social support within this context? (Sources of expertize: organizations supporting burns sufferers, interview with a sociologist about stress and the family.)
4. Mapping altered body image/social support, how do you do this? (Sources of expertize: a clinical psychologist.)

Two group members were allocated to each line of inquiry and briefed by the group chair on the required work. The group was keen to ensure that work was not duplicated. It was then agreed to meet back after three days of first round investigation.

FIRST FINDINGS

Before investigators reported their first findings the group facilitator suggested that people report on their lines of inquiry, whether information had been easy or difficult to obtain. Inquiry team 1 explained that investigation had been difficult in part. While it had been relatively easy to obtain staff anecdotal information about psychological changes following burns, the issue of formally assessing psychological state had proven confusing. There were a variety of tools that might be used to assess patient's psychological status. Some of these focused upon depression, others upon stress and coping. They observed that disfigurement might be understood in each of these terms but it was unclear whether the measures mapped similar things or whether in fact they might all, collectively, miss at least some aspects of psychological change. Emily observed, 'We could read about psychological tests for many weeks and still be left wondering what was most relevant. I think we will need an opinion on what measures fit with this situation.'

Inquiry team 2 had spent their days investigating in the library and surfing the web. They were delighted to report that they had found a useful website for a charity called *Changing Faces*, which dealt specifically with facial disfigurement (http://www.changingfaces.co.uk/). The charity had been set up by a man who had been facially disfigured and seemed to offer a range of practical advice. Altered body image was defined in practical terms here, how people might feel and what it would take to adopt a new persona. There were also a number of textbooks by nurses, doctors and psychologists which discussed altered body image in different terms. While only certain chapters of these dealt with burns, there was a good selection of information about what altered body image was.

Inquiry team 3 had, as they put it, 'hit a brick wall'. They had planned to interview several experts about social support but one interview had been cancelled at late notice. Other professionals apologized but explained that they could not schedule meetings at such short notice. The team had therefore changed tack and used the library to complete a literature search on 'social support' and 'social support networks'. This had proven productive although, given the available time, they tried to avoid reading too many case studies of information. Articles on social support as a process or as a system seemed to 'cut to the chase'.

Inquiry team 4's work had focused on an interview with a highly experienced nurse who worked with amputees. She offered her help when access to a clinical psychologist proved difficult. The nurse specialist had encouraged the investigators to start by making a comparison of burns and amputee circumstances. Both were often traumatic and both were very visible. Both influenced how others responded to the individual, touching, love making, sharing social occasions. Both required the immediate carers to wonder, 'How do I help my relative or friend deal with social encounters?' The team was confident that this information was relevant to the current investigation, even if it did concern a different sort of trauma.

Discussion then followed the group dividing up a large whiteboard into areas for 'facts', 'learning issues', 'new inquiries' and 'working solutions'. The group allocated the following information to various boxes on the whiteboard (see Box 10.2).

Box 10.2   Problem analysis after first findings

Facts

• Altered body image is a psychological experience associated with radical or prominent change in physical appearance or sensation. It may or may not be associated with clinical depression and its extent will vary according to the personality of the patient and his support network as much as the extent or the nature of the injury received.

- Altered body image is likely to increase as the patient goes home and must cope with others who don't understand his appearance. It is therefore a social as well as a psychological problem.
- In practice, assessment of patient's psychological state post-burns is anecdotal and mapped against the progress of previous patients. Referral to a clinical psychologist may provide one of several other test results, typically associated with anxiety or depression measurement.
- Common manifestations of an altered body image include social withdrawal, negative comments about physical appearance or function, concerns about future social encounters or ability to cope, either extreme concern for the damaged body area or conspicuous avoidance of it (through touch or checking physical appearance in the mirror).
- Whatever the possible negative reactions of others to deformity, in practical terms the patient is left with a responsibility to find coping strategies. He will need to manage his appearance and help others manage their reactions.
- Coping is, however, something that immediate partners or relatives need help with.
- Social support can be of various types – practical, morale-boosting, advocacy or defensive (heading off criticism).
- Individuals have their own social support network, which includes family and friends. There are often key supporters who are important to a patient and they may or may not be the patient's immediate relative.

Learning issues

If altered body image doesn't automatically relate to the size or nature of the injury, how do you predict who will need what help before they are discharged home?

Box 10.2   *(continued)*

How do you identify 'key supporters' and what might you
then ask of them in terms of patient support?
What practical measures might help Paul to cope back in
the community?

New inquiries

Ask burns staff to identify what early warning signs seemed
to predict which patients would experience more problems
in the community
Return to the literature/web sites in order to identify practical measures designed to help Paul cope.
Identify a model or framework for mapping social support
so we can find key supporters.

Working solutions

None as yet. But we would like to challenge the group
facilitator – 'What focus should we now work towards – an
action plan, a diagnostic guide, helpful hints for the patient
and family?'

NEW INFORMATION – NEW INVESTIGATIONS

At this point the group facilitator congratulated everyone on
their first round work, noting that several useful strands of
information had been discovered and that the planned additional lines of inquiry were reasonable. He agreed that it was
now appropriate to find a focus for the problem solution and
that this should be to prepare an outline plan of action that
would help Paul to anticipate life back in the community and
coping with his altered physical appearance. However, he challenged the group to consider two questions that so far seemed
under-represented in their analysis:

1. To what extent would any plan of action depend upon Paul's
   readiness to deal with this change? Arguably, rehabilitation

---

Box 10.3 More news

Paul received a letter early one morning- just before he was due to have a physiotherapy session on his hand. 'It's a bloody Dear John letter' he exclaimed. 'Siobhan has left me, she's bailing out, just when it matters.' Paul cancels his physiotherapy session and refuses to talk to any staff during the rest of the morning. He stamps around the ward, angry and insulted by what Siobhan has done. Driven by his anger he telephones friends 'on the outside' and discovers through one of them that Siobhan had started seeing another man some weeks earlier.

Questions

1. What are your immediate reactions to this news and how might or should it affect your rehabilitation relationship with Paul?
2. Why do you think Siobhan behaved as she did? Is this important to your rehabilitation work with Paul?
3. What (if anything) might this episode teach Paul about coping in the future?

---

depends upon co-operation between the patient and those assisting him.

2. Changes in post-burns injury are not only happening to the patient, but also to those around him. How would you take into account the new information provided here (see Box 10.3)?

The group had not been used to receiving incremental information on a case study recently, so this extra information came as a surprise. Nevertheless they thought that this was the sort of rejection that Paul might experience in the future, so it was important to discuss it briefly and decide how it influenced further information gathering. They felt angry at Siobhan's news, not so much because her withdrawal from the relationship was not understandable, but because of the timing of the revelation. They decided that it might have been kinder to have waited rather longer, monitoring her own feelings, and Paul's progress, before electing what to say or do. The letter would place staff in a difficult position they decided. If they fuelled Paul's anger with their own, there was the possibility that he would get trapped there and refuse to move on. Anger needed to be constructively directed. Their next investigations should therefore incorporate discovering ways to cope with feelings such as anger and deal with rejection. It was now more urgent to find any alternative key supporters who might assist him to deal with his feelings.

A lengthy discussion followed on why Siobhan behaved as she did. It was acknowledged that the relationship might not have had a longer-term future in the first place. People who are in unstable or deteriorating relationships also become injured. Beyond that, Siobhan might fear how she would cope with others' reactions to Paul's changed appearance. She might have to deal with stigma, being associated with someone that she considered to be damaged. The group facilitator smiled, and commented that they were making very good use of their reading on altered body image already.

At this stage the group accessed five different practitioners who worked in burns and plastics departments, three from one hospital and two from another. They reasoned that experiences might vary according to site and the range of patients who had recently been treated. One of the hospitals served an inner city area while the other had a more mixed, urban/rural population within its catchment area. The investigators prepared two key questions:

1. Thinking back to recent patients that you have cared for, what, if anything, predicted who would make the best psychological recovery from their injuries?
2. Given the above, do you think you could have spotted any warning signs and, if so, what would that have involved?

The search for practical measures to support a patient was made easier because the investigators had already detailed the best references discovered during the first round of inquiry. Nevertheless, it was agreed that at this stage it would be helpful to prepare a succinct form of record. This was achieved by making notes from the literature/web sites using three headings: helpful measure; focus of action (on what); and rationale. The group facilitator suggested that this was a good strategy and one which might help them identify the most convincing approaches. If an approach was reported in several different texts, then it might be one with greater potential.

The group facilitator was also helpful with regard to selecting a model or framework to help the nurses map the social support

The 'target map' below has you at the centre. Each ring represents a level of support that you routinely enjoy through contact with family or friends, work colleagues or associates. The inner circle refers to support that is constant and detailed. You could say anything here and get a warm response. The middle circle refers to friendship that is useful and thoughtful, but where you would not discuss your concerns in minute detail. The outer circle refers to incidental friendship – a place where people are sympathetic and helpful during social encounters.

1. Write the initials of people who support you and each other into the appropriate circle. Think of as many supporters as possible.
2. Now connect them up with arrows indicating who helps who. Make arrows indicate the direction of support. Many of the arrows may point to you, but remember to include arrows, which represent support between your friends as well.
3. Where do the arrows 'cluster'? Who is really influential in your own support group? What qualities does this person have and how might they help you?

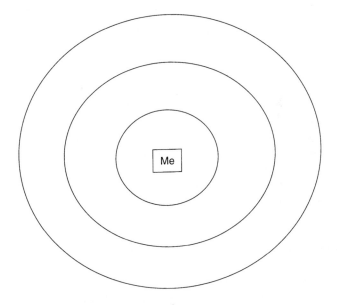

Figure 10.2   Social support network map

Source: Adapted from Price, B. (2001b)

network of a patient. He challenged them saying, 'Why not simply ask the patient – who are the friends you trust most?' They debated that and replied, 'because Paul might not feel like discussing that. In any case, the most influential friends or relatives might not be those that immediately come to mind – they may be people who are able to influence others.' 'In that case', said the group facilitator, 'it may be more fruitful for you to spend your time exploring a tool which does just that. Why not test out whether a very simple social support map might work here?' At this point he offered them the chart, on a laminated board, illustrated in Figure 10.2. As he did so though, he cautioned them. 'Consider this: anything you choose to use has to work within the clinical setting. It can't be too complex or too lengthy to use. Think about whether mapping social support might add something to the patient's rehabilitation, beyond simply identifying who could help him.'

THE PROBLEM ANALYSIS REFINED

Investigators enjoyed talking to the burns unit professionals and reported that their key questions had helped to focus their work. The nurses had explained to them that reactions to deformity might continue for years, so what they had to offer was necessarily more short term. Their experiences came from the first six months to a year post-injury and from ward and out-patient encounters with patients only. Nevertheless, the group were able to identify six factors which appeared to predict those patients who would experience difficulties in the future and to add notes about how to identify these (see Box 10.4). These were admitted into the analysis as 'working facts'. While there would always be exceptions to these, they seemed robust enough to alert practitioners to who *might* need greater assistance.

Box 10.4   Risk factors for altered body image

1. People with limited support in the community – people who lived alone or who were very 'private' individuals. (*Sensed at visiting times, the range of visitors attending and the relationships apparent there.*)

2. People who had burns to exposed parts of the body – they had more to defend or explain. (*Patients expressed dismay at facial burns in particular and distress among visitors was greatest in these circumstances.*)

3. People who were asked to wear obvious devices or dressings to control keloid scar tissue. (*Patients were often ambivalent about using such aids, but still distressed about the impact of scar tissue later on. The double bind of an unsightly support or ugly scar tissue made coping difficult for them.*)

4. People who had unresolved or only partially resolved pain. (*The memory of pain haunted patients, something they freely reported.*)

5. People who fretted, those who focused on their disabilities or problems (the anxious personality). (*Nurses observed that some other patients found other ways to value themselves and focused less on physical appearance as a sign of self-worth.*)

6. People who experienced functional difficulties through scarring, particularly eating or swallowing. (*Patients expressed disgust regarding inept eating or other skills damaged by the burn.*)

Investigators exploring practical measures to assist Paul uncovered a number of problems. The literature authors took different positions on practical assistance. For example, there was a debate about what support should be offered by burns care nurses and what could only be provided by specialists, such as a clinical psychologist or a mental health nurse. It remained unclear what the relative importance of different measures were. For instance, pain management and help with physiotherapy would improve morale and physical function. To an extent this was also altered body image care. Other work, however, associated with relatives and rehearsing life beyond the hospital was distinctly psycho-social. It was not clear what the right balance of intervention might be for particular patients. This said, after much discussion the group was able to identify a series of measures that collectively *might* assist Paul in his situation (see Box 10.5).

Box 10.5   Useful altered body image interventions

Focus on physical care

1. Controlling pain (pain accentuates the feeling of the body as flawed, as embarrassing).
2. Encouraging physiotherapy (mobility increases independence and self-esteem).
3. Making dressings/physical support materials as discreet and natural-looking as possible (Paul might see these as 'props', sources of embarrassment as well as being physically uncomfortable).

Focus on psycho-social care

4. Helping Paul rehearse what he fears, or thinks will happen when he goes home (being forewarned is to be forearmed. Trying out ideas in a safe place before situations arise can help.)
5. Helping Paul anticipate/understand the problems that others might have dealing with his new appearance. (Paul needs to understand others' reactions and become expert in managing responses.)
6. Helping Paul rehearse how he wants to react to social situations, what others say or do, for example, staring. (This is better than reacted 'on the spot'. He may feel more in control.)
7. Identifying lay carers who can cushion the blow, help others understand Paul's needs or wishes before he goes out. (This minimizes the number of explanations that Paul has to make about his appearance and experiences.)

Group investigators described their work with the social support network map as 'playing'. It was an enjoyable form of investigation because they were able to try the tool out for themselves and with friends. They set out to identify its uses and its limitations. On the plus side the tool was relatively easy to explain to others and to fill in. It provoked discussion and this they thought might be useful with Paul, who had time on his hands in hospital and who might benefit from a practical review of other sources of help, beyond Siobhan. There was always a risk, however, that the tool might reveal a very limited social support network and this posed the problem, what could health care staff do about that? At that stage it might be necessary to consider referral to community agencies that could work with the patient.

The tool also enabled the 'patient' and nurse to identify key supporters, some of whom were not a spouse/partner or immediate family member. The investigators made the point that sometimes, acceptable help was gender-specific – with some problems you might prefer to talk to a member of the same gender. Beyond this, the tool needed to be used in A3 format because some of the people who filled one in had a large social support network and the available space soon became cluttered.

With new information on the table the study group now turned to detailed analysis. They agreed that they had a lot of useful information that seemed reasonably robust and that they had an outline of what might be done to help Paul. Stewart, however, observed that what they had was rather 'recipe-like'. There was a need to add in some material on how to pace and direct care. The group had not yet answered the facilitator's challenge about Paul's readiness to proceed with rehabilitation or to decide how to order what should be done first. Carol suggested that these decisions could be framed in terms of three questions:

1. When? (Was Paul ready? Was other care work a priority?)
2. How much? How fast? (Pacing rehabilitation was important, Paul could be overwhelmed.)
3. Where? (Was this better handled in hospital or the community?)

TOWARDS A PROBLEM SOLUTION

Combining the rehabilitation 'what', discovered through their investigations, with the rehabilitation 'how', arising out of discussions following the last round of information gathering, proved difficult. As with other clinical problems, solutions would be best fit. Paul would be one patient among many and there would always be competing demands. The pressure on limited resources, scarce hospital beds would help determine when he was discharged from hospital and therefore how much rehabilitation could be completed within that setting. The problem solution would therefore always include the caveat, 'all things being equal'.

The group accepted that rehabilitation could not be forced on Paul and that therefore the pace of this would be influenced by Paul's emotional state. Siobhan's letter and Paul's reflections on the costs as well as the kudos of a brave act would influence his response to rehabilitation work. Patient mood was a factor that burns unit nurses constantly referred to as a challenge within rehabilitation practice. The group decided that the action plan should start therefore with a careful assessment of Paul's mood, his motivation to work with health care staff. This would refer as much to psycho-social care as it did to physical measures. At this juncture it was accepted that mood assessment was not sophisticated. Only a percentage of patients received, or arguably warranted, a full clinical psychological assessment. In the absence of clear signs of depression therefore mood assessment would be conducted at the 'Are you happy to learn/explore ways of coping?' motivational level.

The solution was additionally based upon the principle that Paul should be taught about the relative merits of psycho-social as well as physical rehabilitation measures. Physiotherapy and occupational therapy were usually a medical 'given', a part of the menu provided by hospitals, but psychological rehabilitation was something that patients received less frequently. The group expected that such work would be emotionally draining for Paul because it might challenge him to think about what he would prefer to avoid. It would be necessary therefore to proceed cautiously. To this end, support mapping would be explained as a way of identifying others who could help explain his situation, his feelings and perspective, reducing the number of times when he would need to explain events himself. It might alert him to other people who could replace Siobhan as a source of support. Work done in this area now might, if he felt able, provide dividends later on.

Group members were keenly aware that helping patients to rehearse what they wanted others to know about their situation, and coping methods to deal with social encounters was a skilful matter. Before they could contribute, they would prefer to work with a more experienced professional. Nevertheless, the rationale for this would still be explained to Paul, emphasizing that while this was tiring now, it might afford him some extra measure of control over social situations. Paul would be invited to decide whether he wanted to explore this work and to indicate how much of it he felt he could cope with while in hospital.

The group suggested that an adapted social support network map would be used to help identify key helpers and that then one or more of these could be invited into hospital to discuss with Paul, and the nurse, plans for managing rehabilitation in the community. This might include asking Paul what he wanted explained to others before he was discharged home, how he would like to deal with questions and whether he felt able to discuss the injury and his experiences subsequently. The chosen helper would then be briefed upon who to contact. As part of this discussion the nurse would summarize to them both what common reactions others might demonstrate upon seeing Paul's new appearance. This would enable the key supporter to understand others' reactions and to help them deal with these before they next met Paul.

During his remaining hospital stay, physical rehabilitation measures would also be pursued. The nurse would reinforce lessons taught by therapists and employ prescribed analgesia to help Paul cope with the discomfort. They would also monitor pain levels carefully to ensure that a residue of pain was not unduly tiring or demoralizing Paul during his rehabilitation. To achieve this, the group proposed to use pain assessment charts that had been reviewed as part of a previous investigation.

VERIFICATION OF THE SOLUTION

Having distilled the action plan for Paul into a series of principles and planned actions, each of which could be defended to reviewers (see Box 10.6) the group then considered how best to verify their solution. Experienced burns unit nurses and rehabilitation therapists were considered authoritative judges regarding whether the solution was adequately focused, ethical and practical. The group facilitator suggested that this could be readily prepared as a short presentation and group discussion that involved the audience of nurses and therapists. If different group members took responsibility for different elements of the presentation and they all 'fielded' questions, this would help them practise important transferable skills.

Box 10.6   Interventions with Paul

Principles

- Assess readiness/motivation first, rehabilitation is co-operative rather than coercive.
- Match Paul's circumstances against those highlighted as 'high risk' in order to assess the importance of altered body image intervention.
- Manage pain and anxiety first (pre-requisites if Paul is to cope with the challenges of rehabilitation).
- Keep Paul properly informed – briefed on the merits of particular rehabilitation measures.
- Proceed at a pace which is manageable and that accommodates events along the way.
- If possible, work with a lay carer (they are important beyond hospital discharge).
- Identify what rehabilitation has not been completed at hospital discharge, and refer to available community care services or support groups.

Interventions

- Pain management.
- Physical therapy – particularly to hands.
- Prosthetic therapy (to help manage keloid tissue formation).
- Map social support and identify key supporter(s).
- Help Paul decide what he wants others to know – brief key supporter on what should be explained.
- Rehearse through discussion with Paul how others might react and why.
- Rehearse with Paul possible ways of coping with social encounters (anticipate situations such as meals out).
- Monitor Paul's reaction, coping and adjust pace of intervention.

The group presentation took place within a seminar room at the hospital and was attended by four burns unit nurses, a physiotherapist and two tutors from the university. The group facilitator had negotiated the attendance of his tutor colleague, explaining this she had herself been assisting a group with a rehabilitation problem in a different field. There was the possibility that this tutor might be able to offer feedback from a different context. The presentation lasted 30 minutes and this was followed by an hour-long discussion about Paul's problems and burns rehabilitation more generally.

Colleagues confirmed that the group had correctly identified the problem-solving focus and commended them on the combining of interview and text-based information in the analysis of the problem. Two of the nurses were unaware of some of the reported literature, but they confirmed that the theoretical points made fitted well with their experience of patient rehabilitation. What was exemplary about the analysis was the balance struck between physical and psycho-social aspects of rehabilitation. In practice, this was often not achieved. By having such a balanced plan the group were respecting psychological aspects of rehabilitation that might prove critical in the long term. As one staff nurse observed, 'We don't see the long-term casualties. I believe that some of these patients become utterly miserable and make their relatives' lives miserable too. Some do try to commit suicide later on, so psychological care is essential.'

Against this, the reviewers reminded the group that what materially affected rehabilitation was the trauma that patients had already suffered and were continuing to suffer as treatment progressed. There was a debate about when psychological shock ended and nurses could appropriately judge the patient ready to hear and understand guidance about coping. Patients differed in the period of psychological shock suffered and in terms of their habitual coping style. The group had not considered coping as a trait, but it was worth discussion as it might help nurses understand patient anger or apathy. Key supporters might provide information about how the patient usually dealt with adversity, as well as review what resources could be drawn upon to assist the patient when he went home. It was important to see key supporters as expert concerning the patient and his background, otherwise the nurse would concentrate upon instructing them rather than listening to them. In practice, many visiting time discussions with relatives centred upon just such issues.

This acknowledged the group solution seemed sensitive – it was not a prescription but a solution that worked with the patient and his capacity. It was ethical because a key supporter was only included in the plan with the patient's permission. Rehabilitation involved a lot of information sharing so it is important to consider who owned particular knowledge and who had a right to share it. It would be instructive in the future to devise research that tested out whether such plans proved effective in helping patients over the first year of their rehabilitation in the community. Rather less was known about patient's needs and progress at that stage of the problem.

11 AN ENQUIRY-BASED LEARNING CASE STUDY

This case study refers to the experiences of practice-based practitioners (mentors) and nurse teachers who wanted to enhance opportunities for learning within the clinical area. The group were committed to making work-based learning a reality and wanted to help students bridge what they thought of as a theory–practice gap. To enrich the learning environment they planned to revisit what had been disseminated about reflective practice and to consider again what mentoring might consist of. When they started their work together they did not see these matters as a distinct problem or something that could be resolved by a discrete solution. Rather, they thought they needed to re-examine their own and others' approaches to facilitated learning, recognizing what it was like to learn within the public arena.

Part of the prompt for this work was a concern that, on the one hand, clinical environments had only a limited capacity for education. Clinical goals, pressures from new national or local initiatives made great demands on the nursing staff (Bleich and Bratton, 1993). On the other hand, students were now being taught large amounts of theory which meant that mentors had to work hard to help learners relate concepts and practice to each other (Goode, 1998; Waters *et al.*, 1999). Nursing had become in their words, 'more philosophical' and they hoped that students would respect and understand what they demonstrated as practice knowledge – that which they regularly used to good effect.

CREATING AN ENQUIRY FOCUS

The study group took a little while to find the right facilitator for this project. Group members were keen to select someone with

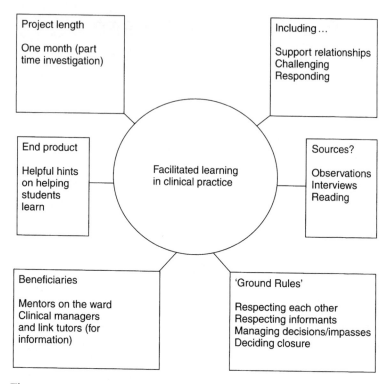

Figure 11.1   Scoping the project

knowledge of nurse education but who did not have a vested interest in the current contract run in association with the university. As they explained, the goal was not to challenge current contract arrangements, but to find a new way of thinking about mentorship. Eventually they selected a nurse consultant with a background in nurse education but who now did a variety of training needs analysis work. 'Wendy' met with the group one afternoon and immediately suggested that it was important to agree the project size and dimensions. Investigations could grow 'like Topsy', so if everyone was to enjoy the work then it was good to agree parameters at the outset (see Figure 11.1).

Wendy listened to the group's description of their ideas and aspirations and suggested (with due respect) that at present it had several possible foci. However, the bulk of what they had talked about concerned the mentoring relationship and different ways of helping students to achieve learning objectives. This extended beyond those formally required within a syllabus to some which were agreed by student and mentor, arising out of observations upon the ward. As one of the group, Paul, put it, 'I feel I want to help students gain something from what they try out in practice. That's something a bit more than picking up the module ideas and saying, 'Can you see this happening here then?' Kate reinforced the point by adding that skilful mentoring included helping students to make sense of the sorts of situations that did not arise within textbooks. There were times when a mentor reasoned through their assessment of what was happening and this meant a conversation about how you eliminated explanations one by one.

Even within the mentoring relationship there was a considerable amount that *might* be investigated. They might consider teaching, demonstrating, assessing, acting at the interface with the university. Wendy asked them, 'What is most fundamentally of concern to you when you assist a student?' They agreed that effective helping, in a difficult, public performance setting was key to their concerns. How did you help a student to learn, when to learn might prove difficult or uncomfortable? The group agreed to distil these concerns into three issues – forming and sustaining a support relationship, challenging students to think, responding to them when they faced difficulties.

The project length was limited by the commitments of three group members who had new projects to start in five weeks' time. Wendy reminded the group that this would provide limited scope for 'offsite' investigations, including obtaining references from elsewhere. There would though be time for making good use of personal experience and observations in practice with students present on the wards. The agreed 'end product' (handy hints rather than a report), fitted well with the practical interests of the group and would probably be easier to write up within the available time span. Mentors were the logical beneficiaries but Wendy persuaded them to share copy with the appropriate university link tutors and managers, who otherwise directed a significant part of the education. It could prove difficult, if not unethical, to prepare suggestions for mentors alone.

SHAPING THE ENQUIRY

At the next meeting of the group Wendy suggested that they tackle three objectives. The first of these was to tease out details of the facilitated learning relationship that they would concentrate upon. There was a need to split the subject up in ways that enabled different group members to make useful contributions. The second objective was to link these aspects of facilitated learning to inquiries that made sense. For example, if the group wanted to know about challenging student understanding, what would be the best means of learning about this process? Who might they ask? The third objective was to place inquiries within a time frame that would permit at least one and preferably two further rounds of information gathering. As Wendy explained, 'if you try to analyse everything in one fell swoop – you get an approximate, rather than a refined answer.' Having agreed to this suggestion, Wendy then invited the group to spend 20 minutes thinking about learning generally. If their work was all to do with facilitating learning, what did the group members think learning involved?

The group made a list of what they felt was included within mentoring (see Box 11.1). The list was not written in stone and the group members anticipated that some parts of the list might change. Nevertheless, it was a list that they could all 'sign up to' at the start.

Box 11.1   Mentoring

Support relationship

- Knowing each other (stranger > colleague)
- Establishing trust
- Agreeing best ways to communicate (when, where, how, frequency?)
- Anticipating how to cope with problems

Challenging students

- Context (when they are wrong/too confident/too blinkered/ too complacent)
- Using questions

- Using evaluation of situations
- Using mentor's own experience (illustrations)
- Reading student comfort/capacity to deal with challenge (timing)

Responding to students

- Spotting student anxiety/uncertainty
- Dealing with requests
- Facilitating versus telling
- Dealing with 'power' (my power to define 'learning')

From their list of mentoring aspects in Box 11.1, it was then possible to plan a number of questions that they could ask their mentor colleagues and/or literature that they read (see Box 11.2).

Box 11.2   Mentorship questions

The support relationship

- What strategies or techniques enable mentors to form a constructive working relationship with students within a limited period of time?
- What are the factors that increase and undermine trust between student and mentor?
- How does the mentor earn the student's trust?
- How do mentors and students agree to manage their working relationship?
- Can mentors anticipate problems that damage their working relationship with students? If so how?

Challenging the student

- Can you give me examples of situations where you would challenge a student, explaining why in each case?
- How do you use questions to challenge students? (What works and what does not?)
- Do you use care situations to challenge students? (If so, how would you go about this?)

Box 11.2   (continued)

- Do you use your own professional experience to challenge students? If so, how and when?
- When does challenge become too much, too invasive?

Responding to the student

- How do you know when a student needs your help?
- What is the best way to deal with a student's request for help?
- How do you decide whether to help the student find his/ her answer, versus provide a solution of your own?
- Is there a power issue in this relationship? If so, how do you deal with it?

The group then identified best sources of information to help them, answer the self-imposed questions. In the majority of cases investigations involved asking other mentors or students their views. Wendy, however, suggested a number of articles that she was aware of which might enliven their discussions. These included material on the following (all freely accessible through the hospital library):

1. Level of learning, deep versus superficial learning (e.g. Ignatavicious, 2001).
2. Reflection and reflective practice record frameworks (e.g. Usher *et al.*, 1999).
3. Clinical supervision (e.g. Sloan, 1998; Jones, 2001).

GATHERING AND EVALUATING INFORMATION

When the group reported back at the end of the first information-gathering period, several members looked uncertain. They had gone to a range of colleagues as well as completing reading recommended by Wendy, but met with a number of problems. These were particularly acute within inquiries associated with challenging and responding to students. The investigators had discovered that mentors were unsure how they challenged learners, or how they responded to students, beyond the obvious answering of questions. While the mentors were sure that they did challenge and stimulate students, they had found it difficult to describe this in an articulate way.

'Why do you think that is?' Wendy challenged them.

Kate paused and then said, 'Because they do all this instinctively.'

'That may be true ... they may be acting intuitively,' confirmed Wendy. 'Is that enough though, if they're working toward particular learning goals? Would you want a mentor who advised you on the basis of instinct?'

The group decided that it would be better if mentors acted strategically. Placements were of limited duration, there was a lot to learn and it was necessary to prioritize what students were told. This suggested a more self-conscious, analytical approach to mentoring.

'Tell me about the literature that you have been reading,' prompted Wendy, 'What does that have to say about challenging, for instance?'

Ruth flicked through her papers and ventured, 'Challenging is all about getting them to become deep learners, people who think harder about what is happening.'

'Good ... anything else?' replied Wendy.

'Because that's uncomfortable and it's easier to think superficially, you have to find ways of pacing the challenge. You can't load the challenge all at once.'

Later, the group described such question and answer sessions as coaxing. In the interim, however, they felt embarrassed that such connections did not come spontaneously and straight out of their discussions with other mentors. Wendy reminded them that mentors had rarely received instruction in educational theory. It was unduly harsh that they should expect themselves to make complex connections without some difficulty.

'Let's do some flow charts on the whiteboard,' she encouraged, 'and use a mentoring conversation to help us fill in the boxes. Ruth, if you act as the student and, Paul, you act as the mentor. Ad-lib this situation. Paul, you want to see what Ruth understands about patient confidentiality. Let's see what is involved in challenging a student.'

The flow chart that resulted from this exercise is shown in Figure 11.2. It was set up on the whiteboard with the boxes and

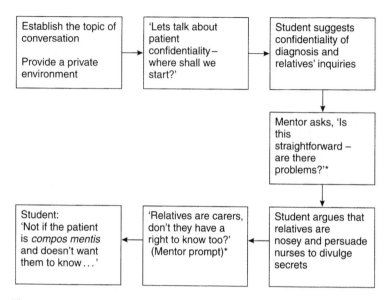

Figure 11.2   Challenging a student (flow chart)

Note: * = increasing pressure, searching the student's knowledge

arrows describing the process first, before annotations were then added afterwards.

The group then debated challenge in the ad-lib scenario in order to formulate a series of questions. How do you place challenge within an educational conversation? Should it come in early or late and, if the latter, what should precede it? Is there an optimum amount of challenge within any educational conversation? How do you know how much is right? What does the student need to know about 'challenge'? Do students always understand what a mentor is trying to do by challenging her or him? The exercise served to unblock the group's discussion. Group members returned to their notes and found examples of mentor approaches that seemed to suggest that challenging happened only late on in clinical placements. The emphasis of early mentoring work was upon helping students manage their anxieties. As Paul later put it, 'We needed some forms of words to talk about challenge, ones which mentors do not routinely talk about. This exercise involved simple questions. How much challenge, when and to what purpose?'

It was agreed that the investigators would return to mentors with new questions about challenging, responding and establishing rapport, based upon the exercises that the group conducted during this their first evaluation of information. Questions were attached to specific educational purposes. For example:

1. Assuming that mentors do not simply want to instruct students during clinical placements, and plan to use challenge as part of facilitated learning, what should we explain about challenging at the start of the placement?
2. Challenging seems to be connected to power – the mentor has more power than the student does. How can we redress this balance so students do not feel overwhelmed?

As group members prepared for their second round of information gathering, the lengthy group meeting had created a series of spider diagrams, each of which teased out further what was involved in mentorship (see Figure 11.3). During the second round of information gathering each of the spider diagrams would become refined. Points would be added about the conditions under which one or other aspect of mentoring work became more important. Challenging, for example, would be understood in terms of the goals being pursued by the mentor.

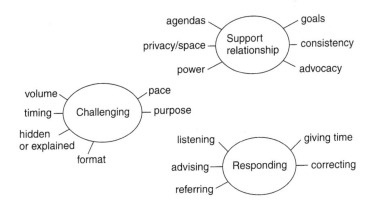

Figure 11.3 Spider diagrams (mentoring)

REFINING UNDERSTANDING

When the study group next met it was apparent that a number of telephone conversations, emails and what they called 'corridor conversations' had enabled them to field a more confident account of what they had discovered. They felt it important to present more and clearer ideas, having sensed that at the last meeting Wendy had been required to direct them more than they would have liked. There were no complaints concerning their group facilitator. On the contrary, she was described as a very analytical person, well able to sort through a mass of information. As a group, however, they felt that they should have been better organized and able to evaluate the information much more as investigators.

Kate said, 'We're pretty pleased this time – we've found some interesting information.' Wendy nodded, 'I'll listen and offer any ideas right at the very end then.' The investigators examining the support relationship then reported first. They had interviewed eight mentors in the preceding days, talked to two link tutors and read a considerable amount of literature on the psychology of helping. While the literature had come from general educational settings (rather than health care), they felt sure that it had made sense, illustrating some of what their respondents were reporting. Acetates summarizing the key points from their findings were presented (see Box 11.3).

Box 11.3   Principles of the student support relationship

Strategies or techniques

- Explaining ward work, describing ward culture
- Mapping the 'ward week'
- Sharing 'best articles'
- Naming the 'classic skills' needed here
- What would you like to learn? (conveying interest)
- My story (include some foibles and faux pas)

Earning trust

- Sharing experiences/secrets/uncertainties (mentor's)
- Observing student interaction with others ('Are you OK?')

- Being consistent
- Being ethical

Managing the working relationship

- Incidental advice
- Private discussions (longer time)
- Appraising progress

Problem-spotting

- Inviting discussion (bigger educational issues)
- Thinking aloud in front of the student ('Does any of this worry you?')

Mentors used a variety of strategies to establish rapport with students, although none of the mentors interviewed employed all of the techniques described in Box 11.3. Successful mentors appreciated students' needs to gain a rapid overview of the ward, what it did and what typically happened over a week. While ward work always changed, there were certain events, such as surgery days, which helped gave shape to what typically happened. Students were then sometimes offered the chance to read several of the mentor's favourite articles on the health care subjects addressed within ward work. This served to reassure the student that the mentor took his or her role seriously and that care was taken to suggest resources that would be helpful. Mentors suggested that students also appreciated it when they were advised of the important skills that they would need to develop in order to gain the most from the placement. As one mentor put it, 'Students come along with dozens of learning outcomes and I reduce that to four important skills. They're about patient education, evaluating progress, working with other professionals and helping relatives. If you can make things less abstract it reassures a learner.' Beyond this, mentors expressed interest in what the student hoped to gain from the placement and 'told a funny story' about their own days as a student, or their first weeks on this ward. The latter signified to the student that the mentor did not think her or himself infallible and promised a sense of humour.

The most striking trust work conducted by mentors involved watching how students got on with other ward staff. Mentors could not control the learning environment, or the student's entire encounters with others, so it was important to evaluate how the student seemed to cope. After discreet observation the skilful mentor might ask, 'You OK? He can be a bit tetchy regarding those tests?' Students described this role as 'looking out for them' and observed that mentors who did it tactfully soon became trusted friends.

The investigators then made a contrast between two forms of support offered by mentors. The first was incidental and consisted of passing inquiries such as the one illustrated above. Beyond that though, popular mentors made separate time to discuss learning with students. Such mentors 'went the extra mile' and often allocated one or two hours outside of the shift to discuss different issues. That might consist of care episodes, projects the student was engaged in, or the development of the key skills that had been indicated at the start of the placement. Less popular mentors limited themselves to the 'watching brief' and intermittent periods of instruction.

The group discussed such patterns of support comparing the merits of short and frequent advice, versus the pattern of passing help and periodic discussions away from the ward. The latter was considered more labour-intensive but professionally rewarding. What seemed key to determining whether discussions were entered into was whether the mentor felt confident talking about 'learning'. This was an abstract idea, but one made accessible where the mentor had a clear idea of the most useful skills used within the ward. Showing and talking about skills seemed pivotal to how important and effective the mentor seemed.

Investigators who examined 'challenge' and 'responding to students' then presented their own acetate summaries of findings. Three important messages appeared to emerge from discussions about challenge:

1. The use and purpose of challenge needed to be explained at the outset. It would not be employed simply when something went 'wrong' but when something was also going right. Mentors made a pact with students to challenge them in private. The ward was a public performance arena where challenge could serve to highlight the student's status, making them feel foolish in front of the public.
2. It was important to use challenge early within the placement and first in a situation where there was something to be learned,

rather than something to be corrected. This said, mentors admitted that they rarely managed to 'stage manage' this to the degree they would have liked.

3. Challenge was most acceptable to students when it related to a specific practice issue. A series of questions about an abstract subject, 'So what happens to body fat in diabetes then?' would prove much more threatening. Useful challenge usually started with a review of care events, led to a general question such as 'What did you think was happening there then?' before more detailed questions were used.

Wendy smiled and reminded Paul that he had used a similar technique in his 'ad-lib' conversation with Ruth at the previous meeting. Challenge questions had been general and became more specific. What is going on here, is there a problem before examining what the problem might be?

Two issues dominated the report of the 'responding to students' investigators. The first of these concerned making time to answer student questions. The primary demand upon mentors was clinical and operational, so they were either forced to offer an incomplete answer, or to encourage the student to talk about the matter at the end of the shift. Neither was entirely satisfactory with mentors reporting the difficulties of picking up the learning points possibly several hours after the question had arisen. The second issue concerned the tension experienced by mentors as they debated whether to tell students the answer to a question or whether to coax them through their own reasoning process. Mentors were less sure how to do the latter and observed that some students dreaded this response from mentors. Students hoped that at least a percentage of their questions would be answered with a straightforward solution.

'Do you think there is a solution to this? Can the mentor expect a solution to this?' asked Wendy. The group's discussion developed apace after this question. Mentors found it stressful to decide whether to 'tell' or 'coax'. If they habitually told students they felt they were undermining educational principles and encouraging learners to treat them like an encyclopaedia. If they habitually coaxed students to reason for themselves, then student questions tended to dry up. Even the most inquisitive learner was circumspect about prompting answers such as, 'Well, lets see what we can work out together' on every occasion.

Wendy agreed that it was stressful, but reminded the group that practice was rarely neat. There were few clear-cut answers. One of the contributions that mentors *might* make to students was to acquaint them with how to manage uncertainty. Sometimes they could obtain a quick answer, but sometimes answers would take more effort. Sometimes no answer was available, at least, in the short term. Perhaps mentors needed to confront their guilt about whether they always met student demands, or always satisfied educational principles. It might be necessary to ask a different question about whether the help they provided explained what learning in practice would feel like in the future, while still remaining supportive in the short term.

REACHING CLOSURE

At the outset of the project the group had agreed to prepare a series of hints for mentors that would assist them to help learners. After two rounds of information gathering, review of relevant literature and extensive discussions, they concluded that they could produce a list of useful hints (Box 11.4 provides an extract). They also decided, however, that they had uncovered several areas where professional update for mentors would be extremely welcome. Useful hints made a number of assumptions about what mentors knew, what they felt confident about and what they understood about students and their educational programmes. In some clinical areas, students from up to four or five different programmes of study had placements. Paul said, 'The hints have to be cautious. I don't think we would say that they are infallible, especially given how long we've been exploring this subject. Wendy, I guess you're going to challenge each of these now anyway?'

Reaching closure after a relatively short project period was problematic. Wendy agreed that she would like to challenge some of the hints that they would produce. However, a more constructive solution was probably to ask the group to verify whether the hints seemed useful with their mentor colleagues. The recommendations for further professional updates could act as caveats to the hints. 'Given that you are assisted with these aspects of your role, do you think this hint would be manageable for you?'

Box 11.4   Extract from 'Hints for Successful Mentorship'

Challenging students

The purpose of challenging students is to promote deeper thought, reflection or to correct student's understanding. You can challenge a student by asking questions, inviting her/him to revisit practice or to rehearse aloud what will be planned next. Challenge can prove uncomfortable for learners however and must be used with care. Therefore:

At start of placement

1. Explain to student the purpose of 'challenge' and why you use it as part of your guidance to them.
2. Explain the formats that it might take, questions, review of care episodes, what next discussion of care planning.
3. Assure them that the use of challenge will not be reserved for situations where they have made a mistake. Challenge will be used to explore good practice, successful care, as well.
4. Assure the student that discussions involving challenge will be handled privately, away from the gaze of the public.
5. Encourage the student to challenge you, your explanation of events or concepts. Challenge should equal scholarly inquiry rather than insult to professional integrity.

When challenging the student

1. Link the challenge to an aspect of care, a specific care episode where practice has involved a number of decisions. Abstract challenges about what the student does or does not know are likely to undermine the student's confidence.
2. Begin with a general question, asking the student to review what he or she has observed, what he or she thought about a care event.

Box 11.4   (continued)

3. Use the student's answer to prepare one or two 'avenues of inquiry', areas where you will ask the student to think more deeply. Use clear, single focus questions about one topic at a time. For example, 'Why do you think it was difficult to manage Mr Brown's dyspnoea?'
4. Listen to the student's reply, watch his or her expression, judging how difficult this question seemed.
5. Confirm to the student what you support in their analysis. Highlight what was clear and incisive. If the student seems comfortable, pose a related question. You may ask whether they could see alternative ways to proceed, other explanations for what they observed.
6. Explain to the student where your assessment of the situation or subject differs from theirs. Explain why you think as you do. Acknowledge where there is leeway for different perspectives to co-exist.
7. Where alternative perspectives can co-exist, encourage the student to ask questions about your perspective.
8. When the student seems uncomfortable with the volume/ pace or sequence of questions, interject explanations of your own, prompts to help the student understand the chosen topic. For example, 'What about Mr Brown's chronic emphysema? I think he has a limited lung capacity with which to use the oxygen we provide.'
9. Limit challenge to relatively short discussions at any one time – they are tiring for you both. Twenty or thirty minutes may be enough.
10. Invite the student to sum up one or two points that they will 'take away' from the discussion. Sum up at least one point that you will take away.

Drafting the hints for mentors the group reviewed what the best format for such information might be. Question and answer format was favoured by two group members, but this approach was set aside because the document became very lengthy. Instead the group settled on three features within their work. First, they would try to limit the hints for each aspect of mentoring (support relationship/challenging/responding to) to two sides of A4 paper. Each sheet would include a brief introduction explaining what was meant by the term (e.g. challenging) and include advice on what could be done before students arrived in placement and what might be done with students after they had arrived. As far as was possible, the hints would be arranged in chronological order. So, for instance, guidance on first challenge questions would precede any advice on closing the education discussion. In that way the group hoped that mentors could locate relevant guidance quickly.

The group discussed the idea of including references to literature on teaching and helping but decided to reserve such information for professional update sessions. Brevity and clarity were what was sought in the hint sheets. Guidance should be ethical, demonstrate sensitivity to student's concerns and highlight the importance of finding a due balance between challenge and support.

Among the professional update suggestions for mentors, the group identified three as a priority. The first of these concerned the preparation of ward induction packs, collections of written material that would introduce the student to the ward and what the mentor hoped that their support relationship would become. While some mentors 'provided handouts', it was suggested that small packs of information could assist students as they joined new placements. The second of these focused upon the use of questions during educational discussions. Wendy advised the group that there was a reasonable amount of literature on using probe questions, managing intrusion during interview, some of which had originally be addressed to researchers (Keats, 2000). There was no reason why this could not be combined with material on the psychology of helping to provide useful in service education. The third suggestion centred upon managing support time with students. Mentors had reported that they were unsure how best to ensure that the students got adequate attention.

Verification of the hint sheets occurred some three weeks after the project period had closed and after the group facilitator had left the group. It was not an ideal arrangement, but the group agreed that it had been a substantial achievement to produce the hint sheets within the available time frame. They felt confident that they could adjust the sheets using the feedback from mentors if necessary. Copies of the sheets had been sent to the link tutors and ward managers by post and their feedback would also be used to modify the work.

While mentors agreed that the hint sheets captured useful information on supporting students they saw a number of possible ways to make sure the sheets had a bigger impact:

1. They recommended that students receive a similar briefing through their module materials about mentoring on the ward. They argued that 'challenge' would be embedded in clinical education more quickly if students started with a clear impression of what mentors would hope to achieve using these techniques. They argued that challenge needed to be 'legitimized at all levels' and from the outset.

2. They suggested that the hint sheets should be piloted for six months in order to identify if and where other adjustments needed to be made. Mentors appeared to see the hint sheets as protocols rather than guidance sheets and this worried several group members. Mentoring was not well suited to a formulaic approach and they had hoped to provide a resource rather than a policy.

3. It was recommended that another sheet be prepared on practice assessment. Mentors were often asked to contribute to the assessment of students and their progress and it was in this context that challenge in particular might be used. Mentors wondered how the assessment context affected good mentoring practice.

Feedback from link tutors proved to be encouraging. While there were some programme-specific comments about the needs of students at different levels and regarding module subject matter, it was agreed that the groups work did represent good practice among clinical mentors. Tutors congratulated the group on tackling the issue of challenge, recognizing that to date mentors focused predominantly upon support and anxiety management. Students needed, and positively evaluated, mentors who were clearly knowledgeable about practice and were ready to ask the student to think about the same. They observed, however, that the guidance posed a number of questions about the role of link tutors. Were link tutors able to emulate this level of challenge and support when they were not regularly practising upon the ward? What should be the working relationship between tutors and mentors if the latter took a bigger role in helping students to manage their learning? They noted that current preparation for mentors provided insufficient information about managing challenge and change and it would be important to supplement this if mentors were to succeed with this work. Moreover, consideration would need to be given as to whether mentors were allocated paid time within which to develop the educational discussions to which the sheets referred.

A folder of feedback comments was made up and the hint sheets adjusted in the light of the responses received. The group decided to write to each of the contributing mentors and tutors thanking each of them, but emphasizing that the proposed sheets were 'advisory'. Feedback commentary had made it plain that others saw this approach as a part solution to the theory–practice gap and to ensuring continuity of education between university and clinical placement. However flattering such responses seemed, the goals that were set out by the group were much more modest. For that reason, it was agreed that they should be evaluated again after six months and that any other discussions about the development of clinical teaching or supervision should be developed in other contexts.

Reflecting on her own copy of the revised hint sheets and commentary from the group, Wendy acknowledged the groups wish to contain their work and suggestions. They had made their intentions clear from the outset, but it was apparent that the initiative had raised hopes in some quarters. Clinical environments were already over-stretched as learning environments while link tutors were struggling to manage the full range of their responsibilities. Tutors had been impressed by the group work, but understood that in practice this could mean more work for mentors who adopted a more minimal approach to student support. Wendy supported the group perspective in a letter:

> I think you are right to resist the temptation to make this project more than it is. The hint sheets attend to the needs of mentors, the difficulties they face while relating to students. This is an important subject and one that needs work doing on it. I suggest that you persevere with that perspective and reassure mentors that it is not the first move towards additional responsibilities at a time when the adequate resourcing of education in clinical placements has still to be addressed. That said, I think the mentor's request for one additional sheet, on assessment is a legitimate one. It looks as though the group might well need to reconvene!

GLOSSARY OF KEY TERMS

CAPACITIES

Nurses, like other professionals, have capacities based upon their education, skills and available time and energy to turn these into action. Nursing capacity includes particular aptitudes for certain forms or areas of care. For example, palliative care, theatre nursing and mental health nursing may require different aptitudes, different capacities. The capacity of a nurse or a team may in some instances represent part of a health care problem.

CASE STUDY

The patient story line or situation used to stimulate lines of inquiry within problem-based learning. Case studies are usually patient-centred. Sometimes the case study is described as the 'problem situation'.

CHALLENGING

Your facilitator will challenge you to think afresh and sometimes again about what you have discovered and concluded as a study group. Challenges are often arranged as questions or alternative perspectives that you might consider. The purpose of challenging is to assist you to develop critical thinking skills.

CODING

The process of making sense of information gathered. Coding usually involves interpreting complex data simply, reducing it to a descriptive label which is judged representative of what has been discovered.

CONFERENCE BOARDS

A part of a web site where participants can read and add typed messages of their own. Communication on web boards or in chat rooms can become lengthy and are usually presented in 'strings' which require careful analysis to follow the dialogue underway.

DECISION-MAKING

The steps by which nurses combine information in order to prepare a plan of action. This may include cue acquisition, hypothesis formation, cue interpretation and hypothesis evaluation.

EDUCATIONAL PHILOSOPHY

The values and ideals which underpin an educational curriculum or approach. In problem- and enquiry-based learning this includes co-operative learning, the importance of inductive and deductive means of inquiry and critical thinking.

EMPIRICAL KNOWLEDGE

This refers to that which is considered factual within the world. For example the ways in which the human immune system fights infection is empirical, it can be observed and measured.

ENQUIRY-BASED LEARNING

An inquisitive and co-operative approach to investigating practice where it is anticipated that there is unlikely to be a definitive solution, but where principles of good practice or alternative approaches to care might reasonably be recommended.

ENQUIRY-BASED LEARNING PROCESS

The process by which a study group moves from identifying an enquiry focus, through shaping of the enquiry to an appropriate closure (with or without report and recommendations).

ETHICS

Ethics is the study of moral action within the world. Nursing practice needs to be inherently ethical, given the nurse's goal of helping others. Ethical dilemmas frequently form part of a problem. There are usually finite resources and multiple demands, necessitating decisions, about who should receive what and how care should be prioritized.

FACTS

That which for the purpose of the investigation you accept is truthful, robust, a fair explanation of what you have observed or discovered.

FIELD TRIPS

Visits to other sites, institutions or departments where it seems likely that interesting and quite often, contrasting, information can be gleaned.

FRAMES OF REFERENCE

The ways in which nurses habitually approach practice situations and define their role. Frames of reference may represent part of a practice problem if they are inflexible.

IDEOLOGIES

Ways of defining reality, what *should* happen on the basis of collectively held beliefs. Within nursing a number of ideologies co-exist, for instance, that nursing expertize centres upon the process of care delivery (rather than outcomes). Ideologies may in some instances contribute to practice problems, for instance where practitioners hold fundamentally different views or where one group of nurses try to impose an ideology of care.

KNOWLEDGE

A nurse's knowledge consists of all the information drawn from different sources that could be used to guide his or her practice. That knowledge which is routinely employed in practice (and found functional) may be called 'practice knowledge'. Knowledge may include theory or research evidence, philosophy and reflections insofar as these help the nurse understand what he or she is doing and underpin a rationale for care.

LADDERED QUESTIONS

A technique for managing the level of intrusion posed by interview questions. Laddered questions may assist you to interview in a more sensitive manner and consist of questions about action, knowledge, beliefs and values.

LEARNING

Learning in this textbook is used in three ways. Generically it refers to the acquisition of new knowledge and understanding and the transformation of practice as a result of learning applied to various situations. More prosaically, learning may be focused towards problem-solving or practice understanding. Problem-solving learning is concentrated, co-operative and inquisitive. It is designed to produce solutions to problems encountered in practice. Enquiry-based learning is rather more speculative, and directed to understanding what is happening around the nurse, why something occurs and what this might tell us about nursing practice.

LEARNING ISSUES

This describes the information that you have gathered but which does not (as yet) fit clearly into the analysis of the problem or situation. It includes unresolved questions and debates about how various elements of information inter relate.

MODIFIED ESSAY QUESTION

An assessment technique which poses questions about a case study scenario.

PEOPLE KNOWLEDGE

Understanding how people frequently feel or act, how they behave in different circumstances such as illness. As individuals differ in their responses to change such knowledge is always approximate, but it often accurately identifies traits, ways in which many people think about a situation.

PORTFOLIO (OF LEARNING)

A collection of reflections and other forms of record which suggest that the holder has learned from experience, observation or inquiry.

PRACTICE APPROACHES

These are the ways in which nurses regularly translate ideas into action. For example, one practitioner may typically approach care in a collegiate way, inviting the patient to review her situation and needs and encouraging her to contemplate what would seem most helpful right now. Practice approaches may reflect a personal philosophy of care, a collective nursing ideology or experiences of successful care delivery over time.

PROBING

The process of asking additional questions in order to understand a situation or someone else's thinking rather better. Your study group facilitator may use probe questions to explore your reasoning and in order to prepare challenges that will help your work better. You may employ probe questions when gathering information by interviewing others.

PROBLEM-BASED LEARNING

A group-mediated and inquisitive way of learning about practice problems. Study groups work towards the formulation of solutions. The approach emulates the inductive/deductive skills that nurses need to develop and use in practice.

PROBLEM-SOLVING PROCESS

The means by which you move from first analysis of a situation to a problem solution. This is usually achieved by cycles of information gathering, information analysis and by the formation of tentative explanations of what is important within any particular situation.

PROCESS KNOWLEDGE

This knowledge about how processes develop – what happens next and about how to make something happen in a particular way. For example, nurses have process knowledge about the typical progression of disease or the spread of infection, they understand how vectors work. Equally, however, a nurse may have process knowledge regarding the conventions of how to get things done, for example, to secure an appointment or to broach a concern with a fellow health care professional.

PROJECT CLOSURE

The point at which sufficient information has been gathered and analysis conducted to supply a solution (problem-based learning) or explanation of practice/situation (enquiry-based learning).

SCAFFOLD

A heuristic tool to help the study group develop a shape to their investigations. Within this text a recommended scaffold consists of exploring practice knowledge, frames of reference, decision-making and use of research evidence within the situation or problem.

SCOPING

Gaining a sense of how big the project ahead is. In problem- and enquiry-based learning scoping is influenced by the complexity of the situation and by the goals to be met through the project.

SEARCH ENGINE

A system which uses key words to search for relevant web sites containing important information. Search engines are provided by a number of organizations that maintain information about the web on main frame computers (e.g. Yahoo).

SKILLS

Nursing skills consist of those abilities to assess, diagnose, deliver and evaluate care. Because of the environments within which we work, interpersonal skills are very important, as are some technical skills associated with pharmacology, medical technology and the interpretation of complex data. Nursing skills may form part of a problem solution, or their shortfall may contribute to a problem.

STRATEGIC KNOWLEDGE

This refers to the insight that nurses have about the 'bigger picture' of health care, the ways in which different factors can influence the delivery of care and health care outcomes. Strategic knowledge includes that which enables the nurse to influence others, to set the agenda and to reach particular goals, using the resources of others as well as his or her own resource.

STUDENT SUPPORT

This refers to the measures set in place to assist learners during the course of their investigations. Within problem- and enquiry-based learning study group facilitators are charged with the support role, although experts or consultants of various sorts may also play an active role.

STUDY GROUP

The group of practitioners who will conduct an inquiry with the assistance of a facilitator. In programme-based problem-based learning, group membership may be allocated by the university. In enquiry-based learning the group is often self-selected.

STUDY GROUP ETIQUETTE

Ground rules agreed within the study group to facilitate the effective gathering and analysis of information. Etiquette is usually also arranged so as to protect the self-esteem of group members.

STUDY GROUP FACILITATOR

The individual who will assist the study group to conduct their studies. Study group facilitators do not solve the problem for the group, but nor do they leave groups to flounder unnecessarily. An effective facilitator is well versed in the inquiry and a sensitive manager of learning and group dynamics.

SUMMARIZING

Periodically within investigations it is necessary to sum up what you have learnt and what you have collectively concluded. Study group facilitators are often experienced in helping groups summarize their thinking.

TRIPLE JUMP TEST

An assessment technique, usually presented in viva form which requires students to analyse information supplied, complete review of additional resources and then present a solution or action plan as the answer.

URL

Uniform Resource Locator – a web address which when typed into a web search or clicked upon within a web site will link you to a web site and its information.

VERIFYING/VERIFICATION

Checking whether your conclusions are correct, or at least, defensible.

WEB ADDRESS

The combination of words, letters and other information that must be typed into a search in order to take the inquirer to the relevant web site. Web site addresses tell us something about where the web site is located, e.g. uk = United Kingdom, ie = Republic of Ireland and may indicate whether the provider is a commercial organization e.g. .com (abbreviated for company).

WORKING SOLUTIONS

Solutions to the problem that you suspect will be useful but which have yet to be verified.

WORLD WIDE WEB

An international collection of web sites and the telephone line and computer server connections needed to reach these. The web includes thousands of sites containing information that may be of interest within nursing practice investigations. The web is, however, relatively unregulated when compared with other sources of information, for instance within a library.

References

Adejumo, O. and Brysiewicz, P. Coping strategies adopted by baccalaureate nursing students in a problem-based learning programme, *Education for Health*, 11(3), (1998), 349–59.

Axten, S. 'The thinking midwife arriving at judgement', *British Journal of Midwifery*, 8(5), (2000), 287–90.

Barrows, H. 'A taxonomy of problem-based learning methods', *Medical Education*, 20, (1986), 481–6.

Barrows, H. *The Tutorial Process* (Springfield, IL: Southern Illinois (University School of Medicine, 1988).

Barrows, H. 'Challenges of changing from subject-based to problem-based learning' (conference paper), *Changing to PBL*, International Conference on Problem-Based Learning, Brunel University: Middlesex (1997).

Barrows, H. and Tamblyn, R. *Problem-based Learning: An Approach to Medical Education* (New York: Springer, 1980).

Biggs, J. 'The role of metacognition in enhancing learning', *Australian Journal of Education*, 32(2), (1988), 127–38.

Bjornsdottir, K. 'Language, research and nursing practice', *Journal of Advanced Nursing*, 33(2), (2000), 159–66.

Bleich, M. and Bratton, M. 'Solving the quagmire of clinical standards development and implementation', *Journal of Nursing Care Quality*, 8(1), (1993), 12–22.

Bolton, G. *Reflective Practice: Writing and Professional Development* (London, Chapman, 2001).

Bradshaw, P. 'Developing scholarship in nursing in Britain: towards a strategy', *Journal of Nursing Management*, 9(3), (2001), 125–8.

Bramley, I. 'A beginner's guide to using the Internet', *Professional Nurse*, 17(4), (2001), 218.

Brookfield, S. *Developing Critical Thinkers: Challenging Adults to Explore Alternative Ways of Thinking and Acting* (Milton Keynes, Open University Press, 1987).

Browne, A. 'The influence of liberal-political ideology on nursing science', *Nursing Inquiry*, 8(2), (2001), 118–29.

Brownell, K. 'Obesity management: a comprehensive plan', *American Journal of Managed Care*, 4(3), (1998), Supplement s126–32, 158–60.

Buckenham, M. 'Socialisation and personal change: a personal construct psychology approach', *Journal of Advanced Nursing*, 28(4), (1998), 874–81.

Burckhardt, M. *Ethics and Issues in Contemporary Nursing* (Albany, NY, Delmar, 2002).

Carper, B. 'Fundamental patterns of knowing in nursing', *Advances in Nursing Science*, 1(1), (1978), 13–23.

Chenoweth, L. 'Facilitating the process of critical thinking', *Nurse Education Today*, 18(4), (1998), 281–92.

Cioffi, J. 'Education for clinical decision making in midwifery practice', *Midwifery*, 14(1), (1998), 18–22.

Cioffi, J. and Markham, R. 'Clinical decision making by midwives: managing case complexity', *Journal of Advanced Nursing*, 25(2), (1997), 265–72.

Coghlan, D. and Casey, M. 'Action research from the inside: issues and challenges in doing action research in your own hospital', *Journal of Advanced Nursing*, 35(5), (2001), 674–82.

DeGrave, W., Dolmans, D. and Van Der Vleuten, C. 'Student perceptions about the occurrence of critical incidents in tutorial groups', *Medical Teacher*, 23(1), (2001), 49–54.

De Volder, M. 'Discussion groups and their tutors: relationships between tutor characteristics and tutor functioning', *Higher Education*, 11, (1982), 269–71.

Dobson, S., Dodsworth, S. and Miller, M. 'Problem solving in small multidisciplinary teams: a means of improving the quality of the communication environment for people with profound learning disability', *British Journal of Learning Disabilities*, 28(1), (2000), 25–30.

Dowie, J. and Bordage, G. 'Psychology of clinical reasoning', in Dowie, J. and Elstein, A. (eds) *Professional Judgement: A Reader in Clinical Decision Making* (Cambridge, Cambridge University Press, 1988, pp. 109–29).

Dowie, J. and Elstein, A. *Professional Judgement: A Reader in Clinical Decision Making* (Cambridge, Cambridge University Press, 1988).

Drummond-Young, M. 'Educating educators in problem-based learning', *Canadian Nurse*, 94(10), (1998), 47–8.

Eastmond, D. *Alone but Together: Adult Distance Study through Computer Conferencing* (Cresskill, NJ, Hampton Press, 1995).

Edwards, C. and Hammond, M. 'Introducing e-mail into a distance learning course – a case study', *Innovations in Education and Training International*, 35, (1998), 319–28.

Elstein, A. and Bordage, G. 'Psychology of clinical reasoning', in Dowie, J. and Elstein, A. (eds) *Professional Judgement: a reader in clinical decision making* (Cambridge, Cambridge University Press, 1988, pp. 109–29).

Eraut, M. 'Identifying the knowledge which underpins performance', in Black, H. (ed.) *Knowledge and Competencies: Current Issues in Training and Education* (London: Scottish Council for Research in Education/HMSO, 1990).

Erdmann, C. 'Nurses never stop helping: caring and contributing don't end with retirement', *Nursing Matters*, 9(10), (1998), 16.

Fealy, G. 'The theory-practice relationship in nursing: the practitioners perspective', *Journal of Advanced Nursing*, 30(1), (1999), 74–82.

Flannelly, L. and Inouye, J. 'Inquiry-based learning and critical thinking in an advanced practice psychiatric nursing programme', *Archives of Psychiatric Nursing*, 12(3), (1998), 169–75.

Foster, R. 'Fertility issues in patients with cancer', *Cancer Nursing Practice*, 1(1), (2002), 26–30.

Foucault, M. *The Birth of the Clinic: An Archaeology of Medical Perception* (London, Routledge, 1990).

Franklin, F., Illmayer, S. and Tredget, E. 'Assessment of cosmetic and functional results of conservative versus surgical management of facial burns', *Journal of Burn Care and Rehabilitation*, 17(1), (1996), 19–29.

Glen, S. and Wilkie, K. *Problem-based Learning in Nursing: A New Model for a New Context?* (Basingstoke: Macmillan, 2000).

Gibbon, C. 'Preparation for implementing problem-based learning', in Glen, S and Wilkie, K. (eds) *Problem-based Learning in Nursing: A New Model for A New Context?* (Basingstoke: Macmillan Press, 2000, pp. 37–51).

Gillon, R. 'Medical ethics: four principles plus attention to scope', *British Medical Journal*, 309, (1994), (16 July), 184–8.

Goode, H. 'The theory-practice gap and student nurses', *Journal of Child Health Care*, 2(2), (1998), 86–90.

Gopee, N. 'Self assessment and the concept of the life long learning nurse', *British Journal of Nursing*, 9(11), (2000), 724–9.

Gordon, N. 'Critical reflection on the dynamics and processes of qualitative research interviews', *Nurse Researcher*, 5(2), (1997), 72–81.

Green, C. 'Nursing and professional negligence', *Nursing Times*, 95(8), (1999), 57–9.

Griffiths, P. 'An investigation into the description of patients' problems by nurses using two different needs-based nursing models', *Journal of Advanced Nursing*, 28(5), (1998), 969–77.

Hek, G. 'Guidelines on conducting a critical research evaluation', *Nursing Standard*, 11(6), (1996), 40–3.

Hilterbrand, C. 'Developing and improving project management skills', *Journal of AHIMA*, 68(10), (1997), 40, 42–3.

Hodgkin, K. and Knox, J. *Problem Centred Learning*, (Edinburgh: Churchill Livingstone, 1975).

Holen, A. 'The PBL group: self-reflections and feedback for improved learning and growth', *Medical Teacher*, 22(5), (2000), 485–8.

Ignatavicious, D. '6 critical thinking skills for at the bedside success', *Nursing Management* (USA), 32(1), (2001), 37–9.

Inglis, S. 'Nursing ethics', *Mental Health Nursing*, 20(9), (2000), 18–20.

Inouye, J. and Flannelly, L. 'Inquiry based learning as a teaching strategy for critical thinking', *Clinical Nurse Specialist*, 12(2), (1998), 67–72.

Johns, C. *Becoming a Reflective Practitioner: A Reflective and Holistic Approach to Clinical Nursing, Practice Development and Clinical Supervision* (Oxford: Blackwell Science, 2000).

Johnson, S. 'Making the right connections', *Professional Nurse*, 16(6), (2001), 1183.

Jones, A. 'Possible influences on clinical supervision', *Nursing Standard*, 16(1), (2001), 38–42.

Jones, C. 'Evaluating a collaborative online learning environment', *Active Learning*, 9 (December), (1998), 31–5.

Keats, D. *Interviewing: A Practical Guide for Students and Professionals* (Buckingham, Open University Press, 2000).

Kennedy, C. 'Participant observation as a research tool in a practice based profession', *Nurse Researcher*, 7(1), (1999), 56–65.

Kershaw, B. 'The long and winding road...the development of nurse education over the past 50 years', *Nursing Times*, 94(26), (1998), 31.

Kleve, L. and Robinson, E. 'A survey of psychological need amongst adult burn-injured patients', *Burns*, 25(7), (1999), 575–9.

Knowles, M. *Self-directed Learning: Guide for Learners and Teachers* (Toronto: Prentice-Hall, 1975).

Knox, J. 'How to prepare modified essay questions', *Medical Teacher*, 2(1), (1980), 20–4.

Koch, T. 'Establishing rigour in qualitative research, the decision trail', *Journal of Advanced Nursing*, 19(5), (1994), 976–86.

Lazarus, R. and Folkman, S. 'Coping and adaptation', in Gentry, W. (ed.) *The Handbook of Behavioural Medicine* (New York, Guilford Press, 1984).

Lobiondo-Wood, G. *Nursing Research: Methods, Critical Appraisal and Utilization* (5th edn) (St Louis: Mosby, 2002).

MacDougall, C. and Baum, F. 'Pearl, pith and provocation the devil's advocate: a strategy to avoid groupthink and stimulate discussion in focus groups', *Qualitative Health Research*, 7(4), (1997), 532–41.

MacHaffie, H. 'The artistry of interviewing', *Senior Nurse*, 8(1), (1988), 34.

Marks-Maran, D. and Thomas, G. 'Assessment and evaluation in problem-based learning', in Glen, S. and Wilkie, K. (eds) *Problem-based Learning in Nursing: A New Model for a New Context?* (Basingstoke: Palgrave Macmillan, 2000, pp. 127–50).

Maslow, A. *Motivation and personality* (3rd edn) (New York, Harper and Row, 1987).

McCue, J. 'Can you archive the net?', *The Times (T2 supplement)* 29 April 2002, 4–5.

McEnvoy, P. 'Using patients' records as a source of data', *Nursing Standard*, 13(36), (1999), 33–6.

Milligan, F. 'Beyond the rhetoric of problem-based learning: emancipatory limits and links with andragogy', *Nurse Education Today*, 19(7), (1999), 548–55.

Morales-Mann, E. and Kaitell, C. 'Problem-based learning in a Canadian curriculum', *Journal of Advanced Nursing*, 33(1), (2001), 13–19.

Morton, P. *Health Assessment in Nursing* (Springhouse Pennsylvania, Springhouse Corporation, 1989).

Moust, J. and Schmidt, H. 'Undergraduate students as tutors: are they as effective as faculty in conducting small-group tutorials?' (conference paper), Annual Meeting of the American Educational Research Association, San Francisco, California, 1992.

Murray, I. and Savin-Baden, M. 'Staff development in problem-based learning', *Teaching in Higher Education*, 5(1), (2000), 107–26.

Neufeld, V., Woodward, C. and MacLeod, S. 'The McMaster MD Program: a case study renewal in medical education', *Academic Medicine*, 67, (1989), 557–65.

Neville, A. 'The problem based learning tutor: teacher? Facilitator? Evaluator?' *Medical Teacher*, 21(4), (1999), 393–401.

Newell, R. 'Altered body image: a fear-avoidance model of psycho-social difficulties following disfigurement', *Journal of Advanced Nursing*, 30(5), (1999), 1230–8.

Painvin, C., Neufeld, V. and Norman, G. 'The triple-jump exercise- a structured measure of problem-solving and self directed learning' proceedings of the 18th Conference of Research in Medical Education, November, Washington, DC, USA, (1979).

Pallie, W. and Carr, D. 'The McMaster medical education philosophy in theory, practice and historical perspective', *Medical Teacher*, 9(1), (1987), 59–71.

Parker, J., Gardner, G. and Wiltshire, J. 'Handover: the collective narrative of nursing practice', *Australian Journal of Advanced Nursing*, 9(3), (1992), 31–7.

Pennels, C. 'The Data Protection Act and patient records', *Professional Nurse*, 16(8), (2001), 1291–3.

Penny, W. and Warelow, P. 'Understanding the prattle of praxis', *Nursing Inquiry*, 6(4), (1999), 259–68.

Peplau, H. *Hildegard E Peplau: Selected Works, Interpersonal Theory in Nursing* (Basingstoke: MacMillan, 1994).

Plato *The Republic* (2nd edn) (London, Penguin, 1974).

Polit, D. *Essentials of Nursing Research: Methods, Appraisal and Utilization* (Philadelphia, Lippincott, 2001).

Price, A. 'How to conduct an internal evaluative consultancy', *Nursing Management*, 7(7), (2000a), 16–21.

Price, A. 'How to conduct a feasibility consultancy', *Nursing Management*, 7(8), (2000b), 16–21.

Price, A. 'Cost benefit analysis', *Nursing Management*, 7(9), (2001a), 25–31.

Price, A. 'Conducting a process consultancy', *Nursing Management*, 7(10), (2001b), 29–34.

Price, A. and Price, B. 'Problem-based learning in clinical practice: facilitating critical thinking', *Journal for Nurses in Staff Development*, 16(6), (2000), 257–66.

Price, B. 'First impressions, paradigms for patient assessment', *Journal of Advanced Nursing*, 12(6), (1987), 699–705.

Price, B. 'Assessing altered body image', *Journal of Psychiatric and Mental Health Nursing*, 2(3), (1995), 169–75.

Price, B. 'Theorising in practice', in Bellman, L. and Price, B. (eds) *Exploring the Art and Science of Nursing II: A Study Guide* (London: RCN Institute, 1998a, pp. 5–39).

Price, B. 'Explorations in body image care: Peplau and practice knowledge', *Journal of Psychiatric and Mental Health Nursing*, 5(3), (1998b), 179–86.

Price, B. 'Introducing problem-based learning into distance learning', in Glen, S. and Wilkie, K. (eds) *Problem-based Learning in Nursing: A New Model for a New Context?* (Basingstoke: Macmillan Press, 2000a, pp. 107–26).

Price, B. 'Altered body image: managing social encounters', *International Journal of Palliative Nursing*, 6(4), (2000b), 179–85.

Price, B. 'Enquiry-based learning: an introductory guide', *Nursing Standard*, 15(52), (2001a), 45–52.

Price, B. 'Altered body image: managing social encounters', *International Journal of Palliative Nursing*, 6(4), (2001b), 179–85.

Price, B. 'Laddered questions and qualitative data research interviews', *Journal of Advanced Nursing*, 37(3), (2002), 273–81.

Price, B. 'Making sense of cancer nursing research design', *Cancer Nursing Practice*, 1(1), (2002b), 32–8.

Pruzinsky, T. 'Rehabilitation challenges for burns survivors with residual disfigurement: promising directions for intervention, research and collaboration', *Journal of Burn Care and Rehabilitation*, 19(2), (1998), 169–73.

Retsas, A. 'Barriers to using research evidence in nursing practice', *Journal of Advanced Nursing*, 31(3), (2000), 599–606.

Rippon, S. and Monaghan, A. 'clinical leadership: embracing a bold new agenda', *Nursing Management*, 8(6), (2001), 6–9.

Robinson, B. 'Infection control in the post-modernist era: immunization and the new public health', *British Journal of Infection Control*, 2(1), (2000), 16–19.

Rono, F. 'A students' review of the challenges and limitations of problem-based learning', *Education for Health*, 10(2), (1997), 199–204.

Rundio, A. 'Continuous quality improvement and problem solving techniques for the acute care nurse', *Nurse Practitioner Forum*, 12(2), (2001), 92–7.

Savin-Baden, M. 'Group dynamics and disjunction in problem-based contexts', in Glen, S. and Wilkie, K. (eds) *Problem-based Learning in Nursing: A New Model for a New Context?* (Basingstoke: Palgrave Macmillan 2000, pp. 87–106).

Schmidt, H. 'Problem-based learning: rationale and description', *Medical Education*, 17, (1983), 11–16.

Silen, C. 'Understanding and qualitative assessment', paper presented at 6th annual 'Improving Student Learning Symposium, University of Brighton, 7–9 September, 1998.

Sloan, G. 'Clinical supervision: characteristics of a good supervisor', *Nursing Standard*, 12(40), (1998), 42–6.

Smith, P. and Price, B. *Research Methodology: Study Guide* (London, RCN, 1996).

Solomon, P. and Crowe, J. 'Perceptions of student peer tutors in a problem-based learning programme', *Medical Teacher*, 23(2), (2001), 181–6.

Spouse, J. 'Scaffolding student learning in clinical practice', *Nurse Education Today*, 18(4), (1998), 259–66.

Stratfold, M. 'Promoting learner dialogues on the web', in Eisenstadt, M. and Vincent, T. (eds) *The Knowledge Web: Learning and Collaborating on the Net* (London, Kogan Page, 1998, pp. 119–34).

Taylor, B. 'Identifying and transforming dysfunctional nurse-nurse relationships through reflective practice and action research', *International Journal of Nursing Practice*, 7(6), (2001), pp. 406–13.

Theodore, J. 'Post-modernism and the transformation of nursing', *Managing Clinical Nursing*, 2(1), (1998), 34–8.

Thorsteinsson, L. 'The quality of nursing care as perceived by individuals with chronic illness: the magical touch of nursing', *Journal of Clinical Nursing*, 11(1), (2002), 32–40.

Tierney, A. 'Nursing models: extant or extinct?' *Journal of Advanced Nursing*, 28(1), (1998), 77–85.

Tilley, S., Pollock, L. and Tait, L. 'Discourse on empowerment', *Journal of Psychiatric and Mental Health Nursing*, 6 (1), (1999), 53–60.

Traynor, M. 'The problem of dissemination: evidence and ideology', *Nursing Inquiry*, 6(3), (1999), 187–97.

Usher, K., Francis, D. and Owens, J. 'Reflective writing: a strategy to foster critical inquiry in undergraduate nursing students', *Australian Journal of Advanced Nursing*, 19(1), (1999), 15–19.

Vincent, T. and Whalley, P. 'The web: enabler or disabler?' in Eisenstadt, M. and Vincent, T. (eds) *The Knowledge Web: Learning and Collaborating on the Net*, London, Kogan Page, (1998), pp. 31–46.

Ward, R. 'Internet skills for nurses', *Nursing Standard*, 15(21), (2001), 47–53.

Waters, A., Brown, K. and Eaton, A. 'Preparing for the future', *Nursing Standard*, 14(10), (1999), 54–5.

Weir, R., Browne, G. and Roberts, J. 'Shadow and substance: values and knowledge', *Canadian Journal of Nursing Research*, 30(4), (1999), 239–42.

Wheeler, J. 'Thinking your way to successful problem solving', *Nursing Times*, 97(37), (2001), 36–37.

White, C. 'The metacognitive knowledge of distance learners', *Open Learning*, 14(3), (1999), 37–46.

Wilkerson, L. 'Identification of skills for the problem-based tutor: student and faculty perspectives' (conference paper), Annual meeting of the American Educational Research Association, San Francisco, California, 1992.

Wilkie, K. 'The nature of problem-based learning', in Glen, S. and Wilkie, K. (eds) *Problem-based Learning in Nursing: A New Model for a New Context?* (Basingstoke: Palgrave Macmillan, 2000, pp. 11–36).

Williams, B. 'The theoretical links between problem-based learning and self directed learning for continuing professional nursing education', *Teaching in Higher Education,* 6(1), (2001), 85–98.

Winfield, C. *Clinical Decision-making in District Nursing* (Guildford: University of Surrey, 1998).

Wise, J. 'Problem-based learning in midwifery', in Glen, S. and Wilkie, K. (eds) *Problem-based Learning in Nursing: A New Model for a New Context?* (Basingstoke: Palgrave Macmillan, 2000, pp. 69–86).

Wong, F., Lee, W. and Mok, E. 'Educating nurses to care for the dying in Hong Kong: a problem-based learning approach', *Cancer Nursing,* 24(2), (2001), 112–21.

Woodall, T. 'Clinical expertise: a realistic entity or a phenomenological fantasy', *Journal of Neonatal Nursing,* 6(1), (2000), 21–5.

Yates, B. 'How to involve hard to reach groups: a consumer-led project with lay carers of people with advanced HIV infection', *Public Health,* 111(5), (1997), 297–303.

Young, A. *Managing and Implementing Decision Making in Health Care* (Edinburgh: Balliere Tindall, 2002).

Zeitz, H. and Paul, H. 'Facilitator expertise and problem based learning in PBL and traditional curricula' (letter), *Academic Medicine,* 68, (1993), 203–4.

INDEX